Budgeting for Effective Hospital Resource Management

By *Truman H. Esmond Jr.*

American Hospital Publishing, Inc.,
a wholly owned subsidiary
of the American Hospital Association

Library of Congress Cataloging-in-Publication Data

Esmond, Truman H.
    Budgeting for effective hospital resource management / by
Truman H. Esmond, Jr.
      p.   cm.
    Includes bibliographical references.
    Includes index.
    ISBN 1-55648-047-4
    1. Hospitals—Finance. 2. Hospitals—Administration. I. Title.
    [DNLM: 1. Budgets. 2. Economics, Hospital—United States.
    3. Hospital Administration—United States.   WX 157   E76ba]
    RA971.3.E84   1990
    362.1'1'0681—dc20
    DNLM/DLC
    for Library of Congress   90-843
                                 CIP

Catalog no. 061161

©1990 by American Hospital Publishing, Inc.,
a wholly owned subsidiary of the
American Hospital Association

Printed in the USA

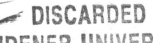 is a service mark of the American Hospital Association used under license by American Hospital Publishing, Inc.

Text set in New Century SchoolBook
3.5M—06/90—0266

Richard Hill, Project Editor
Sophie Yarborough, Manuscript Editor
Lawrence Denne, Editorial Assistant
Marcia Bottoms, Managing Editor
Peggy DuMais, Production Coordinator
Marcia Vecchione, Designer
Brian Schenk, Books Division Director

Table of Contents

About the Author

Truman H. Esmond Jr. is currently the president and chief executive officer of Rush-Presbyterian-St. Luke's Health Plan, Inc. Formerly, he was the executive vice-president/chief financial officer of the Michael Reese Hospital and Medical Center, Chicago. Prior to joining Michael Reese, Mr. Esmond was a partner at KPMG Peat Marwick. He was also the president of a health care financial consulting firm located in the Chicago area.

Mr. Esmond received his master's degree in accounting sciences from the University of Illinois. He is a member of the Healthcare Financial Management Association, the American Institute of CPAs, and the Illinois Society of CPAs. He has authored articles that have appeared in *Hospitals, Medical Care, Healthcare Financial Management, Computers in Health Care, Southern Hospitals, Modern Health Care, Hospital Bottom Line, The Proceedings of the Institute of Medicine,* and other periodicals and newsletters.

Acknowledgments

This book is a revision of the third edition of *Budgeting Procedures for Hospitals,* which was published in 1982 by American Hospital Publishing, Inc. At that time I acknowledged the work of many individuals, and once again I wish to thank all those who helped me, particularly Russell Guerin, who was not mentioned in the preface for the third edition.

The team that put together the present edition, with all the new and updated material, includes Nancy Hehemann and Julie Sacco. Nancy was responsible for all of the word processing and much of the project organization. Julie provided the graphics. Both found the time to help while maintaining a very full work schedule at Michael Reese Hospital and Medical Center.

Richard Hill, project editor at American Hospital Publishing, Inc., provided the necessary prodding but remained patient through my career changes and my many other excuses.

This edition, like the third edition, was an evening and weekend project. Every family member provided the support and understanding needed to complete the project. This book is every bit as much the result of their efforts as it is of mine.

List of Figures

Chapter 1

Introduction

In the health care industry, the demand for services inevitably exceeds the availability of resources. Therefore, it is necessary to optimize the use of resources available and make choices among competing demands. In attempting to respond to the challenge, most hospital managers are immediately confronted with the lack of relevant information about the expected resource requirements, the actual resources utilized for treatment, and the results. Furthermore, the information needed to enforce accountability for variances from expected resource usage or expected results is lacking.

The budget process had changed significantly in the 10 to 15 years prior to the publication of the preceding edition of this book in 1982. It has changed even more significantly in the years since 1982. Not only regulators, but payers, consumers, and other providers have taken an active interest in hospital operations. Hospital managers are accountable to a broader audience. They are also being held to a higher standard of accountability. It is a reasonable expectation that hospital managers should be able to respond positively to questions such as the following:

- How much did the hospital actually spend on the care of the elderly during the past fiscal year?
- How much did hospital management expect to spend on the care of the elderly? Why were actual and planned expenditures different?
- Did increased expenditures result in improved patient care?
- Were the patients, their physicians, and their payers happy with the treatment provided?

The current environment of scarce resources has forced managers back to the basics of good management. Current conditions, however, require that managers be supported with better tools and better information. As a result, budgeting has taken on new importance. The hospital operating budget has been and continues to be the key tool for allocating available resources to meet anticipated requirements and to control actual usage as the volume and mix of patients vary from the expected.

Note that health care must be thought of as a business. Recognition of this fact demands that the budget process include the following features:

- Consideration of long-term (strategic) planning
- Emphasis on sound business practices
- Involvement of persons responsible for implementation
- Emphasis on operating requirements

- Clear description of desired results
- Careful monitoring and control of ongoing operations
- Accountability of those responsible for both expected resource usage and results

The budget should be regarded as a business tool, not as an accounting document. It is the objective of this revised text to identify the essential characteristics of this updated business tool—the modern-day hospital budget for effective resource management.

Resource Management Defined

Resource management is different from resource allocation in that it includes accountability for results. Resources are becoming more scarce because payers, patients, and the community at large are becoming less tolerant of "waste." *Waste* is being defined as the inefficient, ineffective, or inappropriate use of resources. Managers are being asked to justify the resources needed in terms of expected results. They are being evaluated on the basis of the relationship of resource usage and results and are being asked to explain why they could not obtain better results with fewer resources. The questions that reflect this change in accountability, in addition to those listed in the preceding section, might include the following:

- What is the average charge to treat an elderly patient who comes to this hospital for a hip replacement?
- Why does this hospital charge more than the other hospitals in the area?
- How does the treatment in this hospital differ from the treatment provided in the other hospitals? Its length of stay is longer and its average rate per day is higher.
- Are the results for a specific group of patients significantly better in this hospital than in the others? In other words, do this hospital's results justify its higher charges?

Payers, patients, and the community ask resource questions in terms of price and total charges. These questions often translate to increased pressure on hospital revenue, the primary source of hospital resources.

Most hospital managers lack sufficient information to respond to the tough resource management questions. The answers to these and other questions lie in bringing together clinical data (about the use of treatments, therapies, and diagnostic services) and data on the resources needed to provide the services. The challenge of resource management is to improve the tools already available and to develop new tools to provide the required information. "Results" also need to be defined and realistic expectations established and managed. Finally, hospital managers are challenged to provide extensive education and communication to all parties involved—the payers and the community that provide the resources, the managers (including physicians) who use the resources, and the individuals who are most directly affected by the results, the patients.

The availability of this new information will provide a number of benefits. First, hospital managers and other interested parties will have access to information about which hospital resources are being used and about how those resources relate to the treatment of various patient types and disease conditions. Second, the information will contain cost and usage data that relate to actual expenditures and will provide a useful base for comparative analysis of patient treatment both within and across hospitals. Finally, by having very specific patient treatment (and resource) data, hospital managers will be able to account for their utilization of resources by type of treatment, by clinically similar groups of patients, and by type of payment (or by specific payer). Managers will also be able to relate resource usage to results.

Budget Defined

The budget required to support hospital managers in the environment described in the preceding few paragraphs must be a more sophisticated tool than one that would have been sufficient just a few years ago. The **operating budget** may still be defined as the overall plan for the coordination of resources, a plan that identifies the expected availability and use of resources over a given future period for a defined management unit. In addition to a projection of resource availability and expenditure, the operating budget package usually includes a cash budget, a capital budget, projected financial statements, and supplementary explanations, schedules, and exhibits.

The **cash budget** for cash analysis shows how many dollars the hospital anticipates receiving from all sources and how many dollars it anticipates spending during each month of the budget year. The cash budget is prepared by converting expected revenues and expenses in the budget from an accrual basis to a cash basis. The cash budget also includes the impact of such "nonexpense" transactions as an increase in the amount of debt or the purchase of capital equipment.

The **capital budget** is a plan that shows the major asset items to be purchased and the sources of their funding. Included in the plan are justification, priority assignments, and a statement of the impact on operations.

The **projected financial statements** usually include a balance sheet that should be supported by analyses of changes in fund balance and financial position, either on a cash basis or on a working-capital basis. Projected financial statements are included in the budget package to show the effect of the successful implementation of the proposed plan on the financial position of the hospital.

The major functions of management commonly include establishing a plan, executing it, monitoring and controlling activity on the basis of the plan, and evaluating the results. The operating budget is a detailed financial plan that reflects the objectives stated in the hospital's operating plan. It is a management tool for analyzing results and controlling resources. It is also part of a much larger strategic plan.

Whereas the budget required in today's environment may appear to be similar in format to the budget of seven years ago, it is substantially different in its direct relationship to desired results, its flexible application to actual volumes, its relationship to procedure costs and patient mix, and its program (service line) or contract focus. *Today's budget must be a tool by which the senior management and the board of a hospital can evaluate appropriate use of resources in relation to results*, instead of just a tool to project and monitor the level of resource utilization.

The Budget Package as a Communication Tool

The form and format of a hospital's budget package are becoming more important as tools for communicating with a public that is increasingly interested in the health care business. Much information is now available to the public. Third-party cost reports and documents submitted to various regulatory agencies are public information. Numerous payers, payer groups, and employer groups are collecting and analyzing very specific resource data from hospital bills and publicly available data bases. Government agencies, research teams, payers, and consultants are attempting to define patient outcomes and to analyze resource utilization related to those outcomes. Institutions that have borrowed funds to meet capital requirements have made an increasing amount of information available to lenders and potential lenders. Professional associations are requesting an increasing amount of information, which they then use to communicate with specific groups and the public at large. It almost seems that every interested party wants to have a comprehensive health care data base.

Management must be able to assess the community's health care requirements in the context of the current and future operating environment. Those requirements will provide the basis for the development of the institution's long-range goals and objectives. Because the budget reflects the short-term activity that is required to meet long-range goals, it is frequently used for both internal and external communication. For example, statements to regulators and others concerning future action are frequently accompanied by a budget that reflects the impact of that action.

Basic management philosophy is also expressed in a budget, sometimes in the explanation and other times in the nature and extent of activity budgeted. What is communicated and how it is communicated are important reflections of an institution's management. An example of one aspect of communication that still requires improvement is the adjective *not-for-profit*, long used in reference to hospitals. Possibly because the term is not explained or because there is no common understanding of its meaning, not-for-profit is often misinterpreted. People are not thinking in terms of having a tax-exempt status, which is appropriate, but rather in terms of maintaining a zero net income or operating at a loss. As a result, many people do not attempt to understand a hospital's real financial requirements. As hospital budgets and other financial statements are more widely circulated, it will be the responsibility of health care managers to communicate information about goals, programs, and resource requirements (including net income) more effectively. Therefore, a budget is not only a basic tool for management control, but also a basic document for internal and external communication.

How to Review a Budget

Many people tend to be confused by the budget itself because they focus on the numbers (size and variance from previous periods) instead of the institution's objectives. Before a person about to review a hospital budget (or a department budget) looks at the numbers, he or she should understand the objectives that management feels can be accomplished through the resource allocation proposed in the budget. If he or she is not sure what the objectives are, he or she should not look at the numbers since the numbers will not reveal the objectives. For example, knowing that management expects the expenditure for medical supplies to increase by 20 percent tells nothing about the objectives. Without understanding the objectives, a person cannot evaluate the budgeted expenditure. Expecting to tease out an understanding of the objectives through a line-by-line review of the budget is a mistake. If the initial material in the budget package does not describe the objectives, the package should be put away until such time as the objectives can be discussed with the appropriate manager. Once the objectives, the priorities, and so forth are understood, the reasonableness of the allocations can be assessed in terms of the resources required to accomplish the objectives.

Given the logic of this type of budget review, it would then behoove any manager who presents a budget to begin the presentation with a full description of the objectives he or she expects to accomplish with the resources included in the budget.

The Organization of This Book

This book describes the procedures a community hospital should follow in developing a sound annual budget. Chapter 2 describes the need for new management information, and chapter 3 discusses the relationships of strategic planning, operations planning, and budgeting in the planning, budgeting, and management process. Chapter 4 describes the types of operating budgets. Chapters 5, 6, and 7 describe the information requirements at the department manager level, the patient level, and the program (contract) level as well as the basic steps in implementing a system to meet those requirements. Chapter 8 describes the suggested budget process and chapter 9 the operating margin or net income. Chapter 10 identifies the steps in gathering and forecasting units of service. Chapters 11 through 15 discuss the various budgets (that is, the revenue, personnel, expense, cash, and capital budgets) that make up the operating budget. Chapters 16 and 17 discuss balance sheet budgets and operating reports, respectively.

The model operating budget that appears in the appendix, in whole or in part, may serve as a model for the final budget document to be presented to the hospital's governing board. At first glance, the model budget may appear to include too much information. Each of the budget schedules and the supplementary schedules should be critically reviewed in light of requirements to develop and maintain a basic business tool for management and communications. These recommendations should provide individual institutions with a springboard for creativity, not a rigid format to be followed routinely.

The General Hospital mentioned throughout this book is not an actual institution. However, although every effort was made to develop examples of operating revenue, expenses, and statistics that would appear reasonable in normal analysis, there may be instances in which the results would require additional explanation if General Hospital were a real institution.

Because the emphasis throughout this book is on resource management, the annual budget must be kept in its proper perspective as the implementation component of a strategic plan. The plan, including the budget, describes how management intends to utilize scarce resources to meet identified community health care requirements. Strategic planning, operational planning, budgeting, controlling, and accountability for results are all parts of the same ongoing process.

To a large extent, this edition has been revised to identify and address the unmet needs for resource information of hospital department managers, clinicians, executives, and board members. Specifically, it will address the need for, and the suggested process for, developing an updated operating budget that is responsive to the resource information needs of managers.

Chapter 2

The Need for New Management Information

Hospital managers (including clinicians) need new and innovative tools to maximize hospital performance while continuing to provide high-quality health care services. Improving hospital performance requires new information for hospital decision makers.

Traditionally, managers in the health care industry have not related resource usage to patient services except through the use of broad measures based on treatment pricing, annual hospital expenditures, and overall hospital utilization. Communication of these measures has been in the form of detailed patient bills, government cost reports, and other regulatory reports. Thus, the costing of hospital services has been an inexact science frequently biased by the specific relationships with individual users (the Health Care Financing Administration, for example). By providing inconsistent and often poorly defined information, hospital managers exposed themselves to criticism for apparent inefficiency. In addition, hospital managers traditionally have not related resource usage for treatment to treatment outcome. Other interested parties have constructed rough relationships of resource usage to outcome (such as the number of patient deaths) and have used the analyses to question the effectiveness of hospital management.

Hospital managers are expected to allocate resources efficiently even though direct incentives (such as earnings per share) do not always exist. A feeling may exist that the driving force behind hospital activity, be it social benefit, community health, research, or education, provides the necessary incentive to encourage the efficient use of available resources. Noble as these objectives are, they have not been defined clearly enough to be as effective as profit in encouraging efficiency. Many members of the community, like many hospital managers, must improve their understanding of the need for a hospital to have a healthy net income and the long-term benefit to the community that could result from a continuing healthy net income. They must understand what net income is, how it provides capital to the institution, and how that capital benefits the community.

Improving Efficiency through Resource Management

Major payers, including the government, are taking the position that increased efficiency is best attained by reducing the resources available to hospital managers. As a result, hospital managers have had to reconsider their priorities and the feasibility of providing various services. They have been forced to put new emphasis on efficiency. The "stick" approach used by payers seems to have gotten the attention of hospital managers. Increasingly, however, the emphasis on reducing resources has led to concern over the effect on the quality of health services. Caught with poor information to describe the requirements for resources and the quality of service, hospital managers require new tools to analyze both their current status and the potential impact of changing resources, patient mix, and service requirements on the quality of health care provided to the community. A more up-to-date budget is one of these new tools. To properly develop these new or improved tools, hospital managers need to consider several questions.

Who Requires What Information?

Consider the requirements of the clinician, the hospital manager, the government payer, and the national planner. Each one of these industry participants has different information requirements. The clinician and the hospital manager are interested in resource utilization and outcome related to the individual patient, individual departments, and the overall hospital resource utilization by program. The government payer is interested in hospital cost information reported in a uniform manner to facilitate comparisons among providers. The national planner, on the other hand, is interested in social efficiency. Although the tendency may be to focus on hospital resource utilization, the needs of the payer and the national planners cannot be ignored.

Can Cost Be Meaningfully Defined?

The term *cost* can be applied in several ways. Economic costs must be considered in addition to accounting costs. Standard or budgeted costs must be examined as well as traditional or historical costs. As a result, a single definition of cost will be difficult to develop. Consequently, detailed cost information must be collected so that the same cost information may be viewed from a variety of perspectives and at different levels of detail. For example, one view of cost information may be appropriate for a discussion of Medicare's diagnosis-related groups (DRGs). Another view of the same cost information may be better suited for establishing the feasibility of adding a new patient service. Yet a third view of cost information may be necessary when deciding whether to acquire a new piece of equipment.

Can One Develop a Practical Methodology to Collect and Budget Resource Information?

One should note that there is a trade-off between data specificity and ease of collecting, maintaining, and manipulating data. However, it is necessary to measure the cost of each procedure in order to measure the cost of service as defined by clinical diagnoses, surgical procedures, or patient age. To do so will enable hospital managers to develop sound resource utilization strategies and to determine the cost of treating patients categorized in a major program or specific contract.

Can One Measure the Impact of Volume Changes on Resource Requirements?

Since the impact must be measured, one needs to be able to distinguish fixed costs from variable costs in order to calculate marginal or incremental costs associated with specific volume changes, to determine the cost impact of patient-mix changes, and to develop labor and material standards to measure productivity. The same volume statistics that modify (flex) the budget for volume (and mix) changes must be tied to managements' productivity tools and the detailed statistics used for procedure costing.

Identifying Resource Management Information Needs

What then is resource management, and what information does one need to be an effective resource manager? *Resource management* can be defined as the efficient and effective use of resources (as measured in procedures, time, and dollars) to accomplish one's objectives. The information required to achieve effective resource management depends on whether the user is a department manager, clinician, or board chairperson. Each has different resource responsibilities.

There are three issues that should be addressed before a discussion of the new information requirements. First, the resource information in an up-to-date management data base must be related to the basic functional identity of the hospital—the patient. For example, information about the total number of laboratory procedures may exist, but management should also be able to identify the laboratory procedures performed for each individual patient, the date of service, and the physician who ordered each procedure.

Second, available cost information should be formally linked to the services produced in the various departments of the hospital, that is, the output. The total costs of radiology should be accurately allocated to the cost of an individual X ray or other radiological procedure.

Once these two issues have been successfully addressed, the cost of any individual radiological procedure can be associated with an individual patient. Information that relates each individual procedure (and its associated cost) to a specific patient provides the essential basis for management decision making related to planning, budgeting, resource allocation, and other management tasks. *This change in emphasis from the efficient management of a single department to the efficient treatment of a single patient is the most important basic change affecting the process and objectives of resource management.*

The third issue is the need to formally link the individual procedures provided to a patient (and their costs) to the outcome of the treatment. Whereas the methodology and the technology related to the first two issues have been developed and widely implemented, outcome definitions are still being discussed. One category of outcome seems to describe patient satisfaction. Another describes clinical outcome. Other less clear measures relate to the patient's quality of life or ability to return to the productive work force. Measures developed to date (other than death) have not been widely adopted to report results and develop expectations. As a result, most of this text will focus on resource usage at the patient level. Nevertheless, hospital management will be held accountable for results of hospital treatments and must, therefore, take the lead in defining and communicating the appropriate measures of outcome effectiveness.

Developing better information for hospital decision makers does not provide solutions to management problems, but it can help managers become better problem solvers. With better information, managers are equipped to ask probative questions, focus their attention on particular concerns, and become more specific about implementing solutions. The concept of an improved management decision support tool for resource utilization depends on a relatively accurate, reliable, and feasible approach to help isolate problems so that management can implement solutions.

What types of information does management need? Due to the fact that so much clinical, demographic, and financial data are potentially available, the risk of grappling with too many data becomes a definite concern. Therefore, the first step in developing a resource utilization system is to determine which information is most relevant and necessary. To better illustrate the point, consider these questions:

- What is the cost of performing a chest X ray? Is the hospital's staff providing that service efficiently?
- Which specific costs can be eliminated by closing a specific nursing unit?
- What is the impact of starting a new program, such as coronary bypass surgery?
- What are the total cost and the marginal costs attributable to services provided to patients obtained through a new employer contract relationship?

To accurately answer these and other important questions, managers and clinicians require relevant and reliable information at three distinct levels of resource management:

- Department level
- Patient level
- Program level

Developing adequate resource information is a relatively straightforward process. However, the effort expended to develop adequate resource information will depend entirely on the level of information required. What then are the resource information requirements?

Developing Resource Management Tools

Figure 2-1 begins the process of identifying the resource information requirements of hospital managers. The three levels of resource management efforts are shown across the top of the figure, and the types of information are shown down the side. The arrows depict the interrelationships of the types of information.

Figure 2-1. Resource Management Information Requirements

	Department Level	Patient Level	Program Level
Recording and reporting of actual activity	Actual department expenditures and procedure volumes	Actual resource usage and outcome for individual patients and for homogeneous groups of patients	Actual resource usage for large patient groups defined by contract, DRG, age, or other criteria
Measurement and control of current activity	Variance analysis (rate, volume, efficiency)	Variance analysis (cost and outcome)/quality review	Variance analysis/ allocation adjustment/ priority assessment
Development of expected resource utilization	Planned (budgeted) department expenditures and procedure volumes	Expected resource usage and outcome for identified homogeneous groups of patients	Expected resource usage associated with defined, large patient groups (programs or contracts)

Author's note: My thanks to Jay McCutcheon, Partner, KPMG Peat Marwick, who introduced me to the need for various levels of information and who developed this matrix concept, which effectively shows the information requirements at each level.

The recording and reporting of actual activity are historical functions. They tell the managers at all levels what actually happened. The decision support function provides information for the measurement and control of current activity. This information enables managers to focus on the unexpected by highlighting and analyzing the variance between what happened at each level and what was expected to happen. The additional information that must be developed at each level is the planned, budgeted, expected, or standard resource usage or outcome.

At the department level, a manager needs several different types of information to manage current activity. He or she should be able to monitor the dollar amounts and, where appropriate, the volume of activity flowing through each general ledger account for the department. He or she should also be able to determine the labor hours and labor cost and the related department output (the number and type of procedures). Finally, the actual total cost of each procedure should be known, and the procedure cost should be broken down into its separate, fixed and variable, direct department, and allocated cost components. To develop decision support information, the department manager must have access to both the historical information and the budgeted, expected, or standard costs and volumes for each of the measures. He or she must be able to compare the two types of information to develop and analyze variances.

At the patient level, a clinical manager should be able to determine the volume and cost of procedures provided to individual patients and to groups of patients with similar problems. Because patient treatment is the fundamental hospital service, the clinical manager should also be able to measure and monitor the quality of the service. In order to establish expectations for resource usage and outcome, patient groupings for which expectations are established should be homogeneous to the extent that clinicians would be willing to state their expectation of procedures required to diagnose and treat a patient in the group and be willing to state their outcome expectations.

The program information requirements include actual and expected cost and volume for a large patient group, which can be defined by contract, age, domicile, sex, or any of the other available clinical or demographic characteristics. Program-level information is frequently related to the hospital's resource allocation and can be used for establishing and reevaluating long-range goals.

The information at each level is related to the other levels. The detailed information at each level serves as a building block for the next level. As shown in figure 2-2, the basic information at the department level is the volume and cost of each procedure or test performed. As a procedure is used for a patient, the total cost of that procedure rolls up into the total cost of providing treatment to the patient.

In figure 2-2, the average order pattern for treatment of a patient who enters the hospital on an emergency basis and requires coronary bypass surgery but not cardiac catheterization (a homogeneous group) includes between five and six chest X rays. The average quantity ordered times the department cost of $39 for a chest X ray is equal to an average total *cost* of $207 per patient in the defined group. Physicians using this type of information might be more interested in the actual type and volume of procedures used (as compared to the expected types and volume of procedures) than they would be in the cost per procedure because the physician has direct control over the type and volume of procedures ordered for a specific patient. Last, the patient group described for a surgical procedure (coronary bypass) would roll up into the inpatient costs of one or more contract groups at the program level.

The relationships of the information at each level can also be expressed as shown in figure 2-3, which identifies examples of the types of information required for the resource management efforts at each level. Many managers are regularly provided with only a small segment of the required information on a regular basis. The information sources most familiar to managers are the department-level monthly reports showing

Figure 2-2. Examples of Information Required for Each Level of Resource Management

Department Resource Management (Department Manager)

Department

Description	Volume	Cost		
		Fixed	Variable	Total
Chest X ray	17,221	$ 20	$ 19	$ 39
Hip complete	2,503	22	24	46
Pelvis	1,195	19	18	37
Abdomen	4,560	31	34	65
IVP tomography	1,727	120	164	284
Foot	1,761	22	24	46

Patient Resource Management (Physician)

Patient Group
(Coronary Bypass without Cardiac Cath-Emergent)

Department	Average Quantity Ordered	Average Total Cost
Emergency administration	1.0	$ 100
Intensive care	2.6	1,040
Coronary care	3.9	1,170
Nursing—department III	3.1	930
Nursing—department II	2.1	158
Nursing—department I	4.2	126
Theater—level IV	8.1	3,240
Blood	13.0	2,600
Recovery—level IV	1.0	300
Chest X ray	5.3	207

Program Resource Management (Senior Management, Hospital Board, Contract Manager)

Service Group
(000's)

Inpatient Program	Net Revenues	Expenses	Margin
Medicare	$ 5,238	$ 5,006	$ 232
Medicaid	4,190	4,593	(403)
HMO/PPO	3,143	2,989	154
Commercial	7,333	6,006	1,327
Other	1,048	1,362	(314)
	$20,952	$19,956	$996

a comparison of actual to budget expenditures by account. Much of the actual or expected resource information at the department level, patient level, or program level is currently not available. Some of that which is currently available is not linked in a way that facilitates analysis at all three levels. The common denominator is the individual patient. Although most of the traditional resource information does not relate to an individual patient, it must do so if it is to provide linkage among the levels. (It must also focus on the individual patient because he or she is the hospital's primary customer.) A manager interested in analyzing the resources utilized by the elderly population served by a hospital cannot relate and explain changes in utilization to change in the volume, type, and cost of actual services provided to the elderly patients served. The manager is also unable to relate resource utilization to the change in the clinically defined problems of that group, which might explain changes in the volume and type of services provided.

This then is the challenge for the development of new resource management decision support tools: the tools must provide relevant and reliable information related to actual activity, expected performance, and the variance between the two to support

Figure 2-3. Examples of Resource Management Information

	Department Level	Patient Level	Program Level
Recording and reporting of actual activity	• Actual expenditures by account code (general ledger) • Actual procedure-level costs • Actual procedure volume • Actual labor hours and dollars	• Patient group identification and definition • Actual order patterns for patient groups • Resource utilization by patient group	• Program-level group identification • Actual resource utilization by program • Facility utilization by program
	↓	↓	↓
Measurement and control of current activity	• Department budget/actual expense analysis • Procedure cost variance analysis • Productivity reporting and analysis • Staffing requirements analysis • Flexible budgeting	• Patient-specific/group-specific resource variance analysis: —Usage variance —Cost variance • Concurrent resource monitoring • Quality control exception reporting	• Program actual or planned resource utilization analysis • Hospital utilization analysis • Operating margin (or loss) by program
	↑	↑	↑
Development of expected resource utilization	• Budgeted period expenditures by account • Standard cost for each procedure • Expected labor minutes for each procedure • Expected procedure volumes	• Forecast admissions by defined patient groups • Expected order patterns for each defined (homogeneous) group • Expected patient outcomes for each defined group	• Population projections and actuarial assumptions • Cost forecasts • Program volume and cost utilization projections • Hospital capacity plan • Allocation projection by program

management efforts at three distinct levels – the department level, patient level, and program level. The tools must also provide the flexibility to model and change the expected resource utilization to reflect changing priorities and resource availability and to facilitate response to the changing environment in which we operate.

Because they relate to the budget process, the initial improvements to the operating budget will focus on the department level. The same concepts will be increasingly applied at the patient level and eventually at the program level. Outcome expectations have been developed but are not routinely measured and reported for the department level. The current outcome focus is at the patient level. Before long, patient outcome will be routinely measured and reported at the program level. The ability to change focus no longer depends on information technology; it depends solely on the priorities of the individual hospital manager.

Chapter 3

The Planning, Budgeting, and Managing Process

The conceptual design of a system for managing resources includes the linkage of clinical decisions to specific departmental activities and the comparison of actual to expected results at the department, patient, and program levels. Continually meeting expectations will result in continually improved patient care as viewed by department managers, physicians, and senior hospital management. Continually meeting expectations will also result in continually better use of available resources. Where does one begin in order to obtain these improvements? One begins with a plan.

The process of developing a plan (expectations) and managing according to that plan is diagrammed in figure 3-1. Planning as we know it and practice it has three distinct parts: strategic planning, operational planning, and budgeting. In figure 3-1, the first three tasks are part of the strategic plan. Strategic planning is long term in the sense that it defines the institution's direction—that is, where the institution should be many years hence—and its priorities.

The hospital's mission statement usually outlines this strategy in the broadest sense. The long-range goals broadly describe the tasks necessary to serve the mission over the next three to five years and to adapt the institution to its environment in order to attain those goals. In comparison, operational planning is the development of specific, measurable goals that reflect the step-by-step implementation of the broad goals during a short-term period in the future, such as the forthcoming budget year. The budget is the management tool used to allocate the resources to those responsible in order to attain the specific goals in the operating plan. Throughout management history, the challenge has been to maintain linkage from the strategy to the operating plan to the budget such that one can directly relate the appropriate use of resources by specific managers to the attainment of operating objectives and, over a course of several years, to the attainment of long-term goals.

The planning, budgeting, and managing process begins with a statement of the hospital's mission. This statement points the direction for all activity, gives the activity purpose, and establishes a very high-level goal. In basic terms, the mission of a hospital might be to improve the overall health status of the community through the provision of high-quality hospital service at a reasonable cost and to contribute to the overall improvement in the delivery of care through the support of appropriate research and education. The actual statement would be more specific, but even in this example, the focus is clearly on the care of the patient.

Figure 3-1. The Planning, Budgeting, and Managing Process

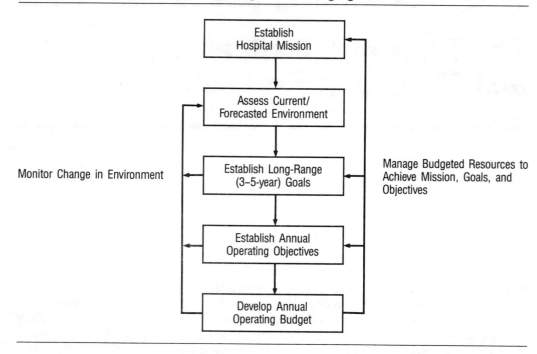

The next step in the process is environmental assessment of the hospital. The assessment describes the conditions under which the hospital managers expect to conduct their business during the period covered by the plan, probably three to five years. As expected, it is somewhat more specific about forecasts for the near future than for the fifth year of a five-year plan.

The goal statements are generally longer term—what is to be accomplished over the three- to five-year period? The statements are specific enough, however, to provide a measurement for successfully attaining each individual goal. The annual operating objectives are the specific, measurable objectives assigned to specific managers and given a specific deadline date.

The goal statements and the objectives are typically program oriented and defined in clinical terms. This is understandable given the nature of the mission and the goals, which focus on community health in general and patient care in specific. Goal statements and objectives are also prioritized. Given the hospital's limited resources, some programs and their related goals and objectives will have priority over others. Because goals or objectives are not expressed in dollar amounts, they are typically not financial in nature.

The annual operating budget is the management tool that is used to allocate the resources to accomplish the operating objectives. Whereas the objectives are program oriented, the budget has typically been department oriented. The operating objectives are developed from the top down from the mission statement, the environmental assessment, and the long-range goals, but the annual budget has typically been developed from the bottom up, with the department managers submitting resource requirements expressed in terms of staffing and dollar requirements that are rolled up to determine total hospital requirements. During the course of the year, resources are managed according to the budget, and usage is measured and reported every month or every four weeks.

Linking the Budget to Long-Term Goals

The key to linking the budget to strategic long-term goals is an effective annual operating plan. Matching resources against the operating plan forms the basis of the annual operating budget. The annual budget can still be department based, but it must be program oriented.

A coordinated process of strategic and operational planning and budgeting is necessary to effectively focus and utilize scarce resources over a long period of time. Establishing strategy is the joint responsibility of a hospital's governing board and senior management. Strategic planning is the responsibility of senior management, with review and approval by the governing board (see figure 3-2). The development of strategic plans is a top–down process.

In contrast, the development of specific operational plans consistent with broad goals and policies is a bottom–up process. The operational plan is the responsibility of line management, with the direct involvement of department directors and other responsibility center managers. Senior management reviews and approves the operational plans developed by line management. This activity and the budget process are interrelated. The budget may be viewed as the operational plan expressed in terms of dollars.

The planning, budgeting, and managing process is theoretically sound, but it typically breaks down when managers attempt to relate the operating objectives to the operating budget. In actual practice, the resource allocations in the department budget cannot be identified with the programmatic planning objectives, which cross several or many departments. It is the objective of this text to describe why and how these two functions can be made to work together to link strategy to resource allocation and control.

Establishing the Planning Process

Plans exist for all institutions; most are very general, and many have not been recorded in a single document. As the formal planning process begins at each institution, it is expected that the result of the first year's planning cycle will be of a general nature. However, as experience is accumulated with specific goal-oriented planning and with information from the evaluation process, subsequent cycles will become more detailed and the process itself will be modified. Although the specific techniques of management by objectives or zero-based budgeting may not be adopted by the institution, their methodologies, like the planning process, are goal oriented, and their basic concepts will naturally find their way into the process.

The evolution of the planning and budgeting process promotes a more systematic method of management reporting and accountability at all levels. It also produces a unified and clearly understood frame of reference for future planning and budgeting. Ultimately, the process should strengthen management's ability to anticipate and respond to situations in an increasingly complex and regulatory environment and to further public understanding and acceptance of the institution's role in the community.

Strategic Planning

Strategic planning is defined by the American Hospital Association in the publication *Environmental Assessment of the Hospital Industry 1979* (Chicago, 1979), which is a summary of its own corporate planning. When the word *institution* is substituted

Figure 3-2. Responsibility for, and Relationship of, Planning and Budgeting

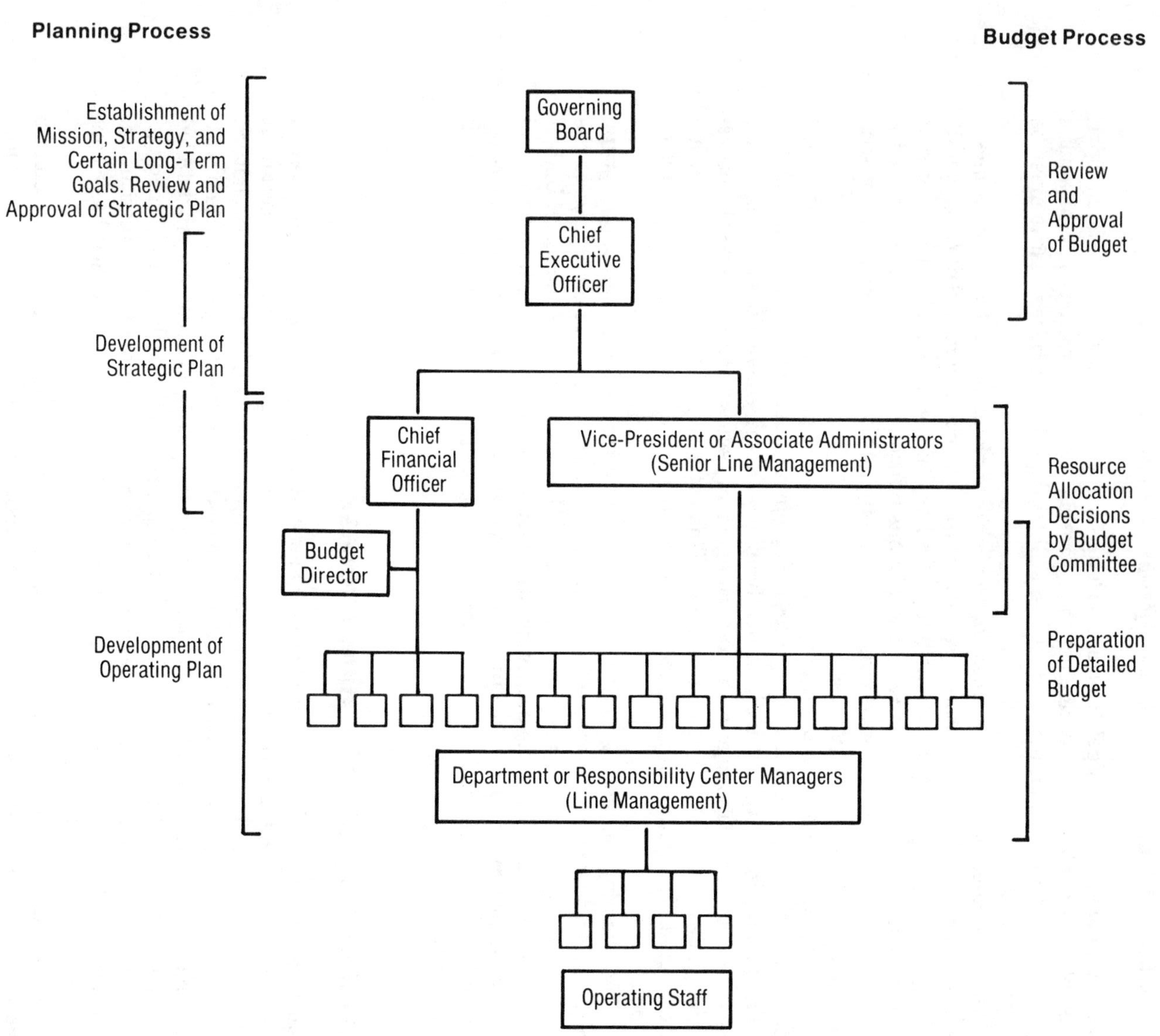

for the word *Association*, the definition reads as follows: "Strategic planning is the process of determining the overall direction in which the institution will be moving in the future. . . . The result of this process is a corporate strategy that states succinctly the objectives of the institution along with the nature and scope of emphasis that will be given to each major program area within the institution" (p. 41).

A statement of institutional strategy should be preceded by an environmental analysis, a descriptive analysis of the institution, and the environment in which the institution operates. This description makes certain assumptions regarding future environmental changes, analyzes their possible impact on the types and amounts of resources, and evaluates the institution's capacity to respond to the environmental implications. These assumptions consider events that are anticipated during the period covered by the strategic plan (the forthcoming three to five years). Some institutions may find it appropriate to include portions of the environmental analysis in the narrative sections of the budget package.

All of the following features should be included in the institution's environmental analysis:

- *Description of the service area:* A description of the geographic distribution of patients and referral patterns; transportation available in the area for access to the hospital; age, social, ethnic, and economic mix of the service area's population and related trends; and other major sources of health care delivery in the area.
- *Analysis of services offered (by location):* A breakdown of beds by service for the most recent three years; a description of ambulatory services offered during the same period; and statistical information for each offered service that shows admissions, average length of stay, patient days, and average available beds for the past three years. As hospitals expand to multilocation providers, the information should be shown by location in order to relate services to the description of the service area. Where the information is available, it would be very helpful to show the statistics for the most significant programs, as defined by clinical groupings, medical staff organization, or the Medicare diagnosis-related groups (DRGs). The program definitions should follow the programs that are most often utilized in the hospital's planning process.
- *Description of medical staff:* A breakdown by specialty, average age by specialty, and identification of major admitting physicians or group practices. Where the information is available, the medical staff analysis should contain a programmatic breakdown of the patients admitted by major admitting physicians. The analysis for each physician should identify such summary information as the admissions, patient days, average length of stay, gross charges, payer mix, and relative profitability (gross margin) by programmatic patient groups.
- *Description of physical plant:* The location of the facility; a brief description of each building, including information on its age and operating deficiencies (if any); and an analysis of potential use of the surrounding area for expansion.
- *Assessment of quality of service:* Accreditations; significant comments from the most recent survey by the Joint Commission on Accreditation of Healthcare Organizations; results of patient, physician, and nurse surveys; and a description of educational affiliations. As quality assurance or quality improvement programs are instituted, this section should include more customer satisfaction information and substantial information describing the treatment outcome for specific significant patient groups.
- *Assessment of employee relations:* The status of union or other bargaining unit agreements, an analysis of vacant positions and reasons for difficulty in filling the positions, a general description of wage scales relative to other opportunities

in the community, and such statistics as number of employees by employee classification over the past three years and employees per equivalent occupied bed during the same period.

- *Assessment of financial position:* Comparative financial statements covering the past three years, analysis of payer mix for all patients during the same period, comparison of basic daily charges (room rates) for hospitals in the community or service area, and a description of significant (or limiting) debt covenants (if any).
- *Descriptions of relevant community organizations and appropriate governmental regulatory bodies:*
  - Community groups: A description of active local community organizations and the hospital's relationships with them
  - Local and state regulatory bodies: A description of the scope of activity and the major emphasis of local and state planning agencies, the hospital's relationship with local government, and the status of coverage and payment terms offered by state third-party payers
  - Federal agencies: An analysis of the current status of regulations that affect the hospital as well as an analysis of the impact of specific pending legislation and regulations

Examples of assumptions in several different categories that may be included in the description of an institution's environment include the following:

- *Population and disease trends:* "Nationally, as well as locally, the proportion of the population over age 65 will increase. In 1980, 24,900,000 persons, or 11.2 percent of the total population, were 65 years or older. Those statistics will be 29,800,000 (12.2 percent) by 1990 and 45,100,000 (15.5 percent) by the year 2020. In this service area, it is estimated that by 1995 one of every five persons will be 65 years old or older. As a result, health care institutions, particularly those in this area, will face increasing demands for services related to the chronic illnesses of a geriatric population."
- *Public attitude:* "As the premiums for traditional insurance plans surpassed the premiums for capitation plans, business and labor leaders have accorded alternative delivery mechanisms (such as preferred provider organizations) greater credibility as cost-containment devices and will more aggressively promote these alternatives. The Metropolitan Business Group, which includes most of the major employers in the community, has formed a preferred provider organization for the purpose of selective contracting with health care providers."
- *State regulation:* "The state contract care system currently being developed for the state's Medicaid program will go into effect during 1991 and will be used to set this hospital's rates for the fiscal year beginning 1992. The 'suggested' contract rates will likely be established on the basis of 1989 costs."

The entire environmental analysis should clearly reflect the relative strengths and weaknesses of the hospital because the analysis must form the basis for the formulation of realistic strategic goals and objectives.

In addition to the environmental analysis, the strategic plan should include the following four elements:

- Mission statement
- Statement of principles and management philosophy and policy
- Goals
- Objectives

The mission statement is a relatively short description (perhaps several paragraphs) of the hospital's role and purpose in broad terms. The statement should describe the hospital's line of business and its intended market as well as the community-related goals of senior management and the governing board. The hospital's charter has the basic elements of such a statement but must be expanded to provide a general direction for the future development of the institution.

Statements of principles and management philosophy and policy are extensions of the mission statement. They guide management behavior and form the parameters for the development of the hospital's strategic and operational objectives. As an example, a policy may be stated as follows: "Hospital management should be guided first and foremost by the needs of the patients, be responsive to the health care needs of the community, ensure that care is provided in a humane and sensitive manner, and foster effectiveness, efficiency, and financial strength."

Hospital goals are statements that describe a strategic position to be attained or a purpose to be achieved by the hospital. Together, goals describe what hospital management wants to accomplish during the period covered by the strategic plan. Hospital goals provide uniform direction to the objective setting, operational planning, and budgeting process. The following is an example of a hospital goal: "In order to meet the needs of the aging population in our community, General Hospital will develop a comprehensive program to provide effective diagnosis and treatment of diseases associated with aging and related rehabilitation." Goal implementation usually takes a long time.

Hospital objectives are statements of the specific desired results the hospital should achieve during a specific period. These results must be related to the goal statements. Objectives should be measurable and attainable during either a long-term or short-term period. Strategic objectives are long term, whereas operating objectives are short term to coincide with achievements desired within the budget period. A statement of an objective should include, where possible and appropriate, the following elements:

- *What:* A description of the situation or condition to be achieved upon completion of the objective
- *How much:* The level of accomplishment, that is, a quantified description of the situation or condition to be attained
- *Who:* The particular target population or portion of the environment that will be affected by the achievement
- *Where:* The geographic area to be included in the program
- *When:* The time by which the desired situation or condition should be attained

For example, the following could be a statement of a strategic objective: "By 1993, the hospital shall complete the renovations necessary to make the west wing of the hospital fully operational as a facility for the chronically ill elderly and as an extended care facility for the elderly, with a balance between general and selected care programs for elderly patients who have previously diagnosed chronic diseases."

As is obvious in this example, the strategic objective is still somewhat broad. A single person is not responsible for its successful completion. Rather, the senior management and the hospital board are collectively responsible. The objective does not delineate the steps by which the results will be accomplished or who will be responsible. Even though the objective is broad, its long-term accomplishment can and should be broken down into short-term objectives, which are included in the operational plan and expressed in monetary terms in the budget. The next step in the planning process, therefore, is the development of an operational plan.

Operational Planning and Budgeting

Operational planning and budgeting are the processes through which corporate strategy is implemented. Assuming that the strategic plan covers the forthcoming three years, the strategic objectives will describe the condition, situation, or level of achievement to be reached at the end of the three-year period. The overall result is the attainment of the goals as stated in the strategic plan. The activity necessary in the first year to attain the strategic objectives by the end of the third year is expressed in the current operating plan. The operating plan translated into dollars is the budget. Operating plans for future years should also be accompanied by projections of the general financial requirements.

These plans form the basis of a long-range financial forecast. The following may be an operational objective for 1992: "By the beginning of fiscal year 1993, the hospital shall recruit 54 registered nurses who are committed to the care of the elderly to staff the geriatric facility." The budget for 1992 would contain the cost of recruiting the nurses. Because the longer-term objective was to have the geriatric facility in the west wing fully operational by 1993 (assuming that the shorter-term goals for renovation and staffing are attained), the budget for fiscal 1993 would contain the salary and fringe benefits of 54 nurses along with all the other costs of operating the geriatric facility. This objective would be listed as one of several activities expected of a given department manager so that it is clear from the document who is responsible for recruiting the nurses.

Restated, the two results of the operational planning and budgeting process are:

- An operating plan that states specific objectives for a one-year period for each responsibility center or appropriate organizational group of centers
- A budget that identifies the specific activities required to carry out the operating plan and the resources required for those activities

Management Control and the Budgeting and Planning Process

As historically defined, a budget might focus only on the responsibility and resources of each department manager separately. The department budgets are appropriate because, as shown in the example of the geriatric facility, a department manager will be responsible for staffing the facility. But what about the person who has the responsibility for the overall geriatric program?

During the course of determining the need and planning for a special geriatric facility, the needs of the community were carefully examined, physician referral patterns and current admitting and utilization patterns were analyzed, and the impact on all major diagnostic and treatment departments in the hospital was projected. Is it not appropriate to develop a program budget for the person managing the geriatric program that would identify the volume and type of patients expected to use the facility and the hospital resources that those patients would be expected to consume? The program budget would serve the program manager, just as the department budget serves the department manager, in monitoring and controlling resources during the budget year. Comparisons and analyses of the program budget versus actual results during the year would also help the department manager better understand, and anticipate, changes in demand for department services.

The planning and budgeting processes together with the process of management control are ongoing because changes in the internal and external environment are continuous. Figure 3-3 illustrates the components of this ongoing process: accumulating and analyzing information about the environment, reassessing the current status of the institution, and identifying assumptions regarding the future. In turn, long-term goals are reevaluated and priorities are revised as necessary. The results of these efforts are compared with goals and long-term objectives at the same time that they are

Figure 3-3. Continuous Cycles of Planning, Budgeting, and Control

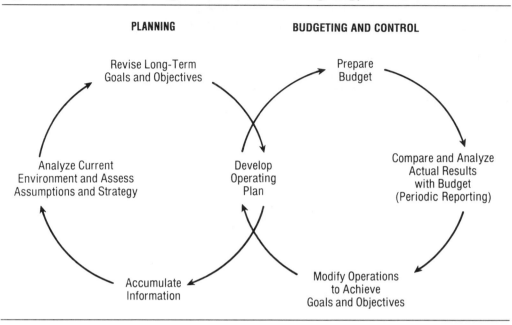

reviewed against the operating plan's short-term objectives, which are the incremental steps within the scope of the long-range objectives. Based on this review, a new operating plan is developed, which establishes priorities, directions, and levels of achievement for the next year. The operating plan, which provides the link between the longer-term strategy and the operating budget, is translated into department and program budgets. The budgeted activity and resource utilization are measured monthly against actual results as a part of the hospital's responsibility reporting system. The results are analyzed against the operational objectives, and if necessary, adjustments are made in operations to achieve the objectives. The cycles overlap and continue.

Budget Period

Traditionally, the preparation of a budget is an annual process, and the budget prepared covers one year. It is difficult to develop a budget that is based on program strategy when the focus is only on one year. An operating plan that breaks longer-term goals into year-by-year objectives facilitates the preparation of an annual budget, but a much-improved annual budget would result from a focus that includes more than one year. Just as operating plans cover more than one year (with a set of objectives for each of several years) to guide the accomplishment of longer-term goals, a budget should also cover several years to show how resources will be allocated to accomplish the objectives.

An up-to-date budget process should include the preparation of budgets for the next two years. This longer view facilitates program thinking and allows managers to visualize and allocate resources to accomplish longer-term goals. Basically, following the thinking and the process identified in this text, management should develop a detailed budget for the next fiscal year and a more general budget that follows the operating plan for the next fiscal year (two fiscal years hence). The process of developing each year's detailed budget is made easier by the availability of the second year's budget. The assumptions used in preparation of the second year's budget are reviewed in relation to an updated environmental analysis and operating plan. The second year's budget is then expanded in terms of detail to become the next year's budget and a new second year's budget is prepared.

As noted in this text, the planning, budgeting, and managing process is continuous. To facilitate that continuity, the budget should be a continuing process with a longer-term emphasis. It should not be a jerky, stop/start annual process that focuses only on the next 12 months. A two-year budget will help to facilitate longer-term thinking and to better integrate the resource allocation process into the planning process.

Chapter 4

Operating Budget

Based on the preceding chapters, it must appear to the reader that this text is describing an operating budget substantially different from that described in the earlier edition of this book as well as from the budget package currently found in most hospitals. Such an observation is true! Management requirements have changed. Fortunately, data availability and technology have improved to support more sophisticated management information requirements and to support a more up-to-date planning, budgeting, and managing process.

Management has more control over some phases of the previously defined cycles of planning and budgeting than over others. For example, although managers react to the environment, they can change it only slightly. Analyzing and assessing the environment, anticipating change, and establishing long-range goals are the responsibilities of top-level management. This process is not only the most difficult but also the most critical part of management. Decisions regarding long-range goals are often made without enough knowledge of the future to predict the results. This is particularly true as a result of recent changes in the environment in which hospitals operate. However, a better understanding of the future can be developed from a better understanding of the hospital and its environment as they currently exist. This understanding of why events and outcomes occur is necessary for building a solid platform on which to establish direction and expectations for the future. Once the overall direction of the institution has been established, it cannot be changed quickly or easily.

On the other hand, decisions in the operating plan or budget cycle cover a shorter term and are goal oriented, with specific levels of attainment. Therefore, responsibility within this cycle is controllable, and budgets and objectives that can be and will be achieved can be developed. Information systems that identify how well management is controlling the achievement of objectives can also be developed. Information systems that support sophisticated gathering and analysis of relevant data are available. Systems support is also available to communicate objectives and to monitor how well managers at the department level, the patient level, and the program level are controlling the achievement of these objectives.

It is important to understand the interrelationship of the strategic planning cycle and the control cycle of operational planning and budgeting. Assumptions must be made regarding management's ability to achieve short-term objectives that are based on long-term goals. Long-term goals were in turn developed from the assessment of the current environment and anticipated future events over which management has little or no control. The strategic plan will change with time and circumstances and will be different for each institution. Just as there is no right or perfect plan, there is no right or perfect budget or perfect process with which to develop one. It is possible, however, to illustrate approaches and suggest guidelines to follow in the budget process. This chapter and the rest of the book offer several approaches to developing the required budget tools and some guidelines that can be easily adapted to fit the unique circumstances, plans, and characteristics of an institution.

Components of the Operating Budget

The basic component of an up-to-date operating budget is data—a great deal of clinical and financial data. The data can be used to focus on a department or on a program, but the common focus for most of the data is on the patients treated by the hospital. It is the objective of the planning and budgeting process to gather and understand the data, to turn them into useful information, and to construct tools from them to guide the hospital toward attainment of its mission. It is the objective of the managing process to monitor and control the utilization of available resources in order to meet the objectives established in the planning and budgeting process.

The basic objectives of the operating budget process are to develop a document that:

- Defines in statistical and monetary terms the operating plans of the hospital
- Describes the allocation of available resources for most effectively attaining the objectives in the operating plan
- Provides a basis for evaluating the financial performance of the plans
- Provides a useful tool for the control of costs
- Presents a tool for communicating short-range plans and financial requirements both within the organization and to the hospital's community

In addition to a summary of the hospital's strategy and long-term goals, the operating budget package should include the following elements:

- Flexible revenue and expense budget
- Program budget (for individual significant programs)
- Cash budget
- Capital budget
- Projected balance sheet and related statements
- Supplementary explanations, schedules, and exhibits to explain assumptions, analyze change from period to period, and provide additional detail where appropriate

The flexible **revenue budget** and **expense budget** include estimates of gross patient revenue; allowances for cost-based payers and uncollectible accounts; expenses for personnel, supplies, depreciation, interest, and insurance; and other non–patient care operating and nonoperating revenue and expenses. The revenue and expense budget also includes statistical estimates for occupancy (patient days), patient mix, specific ancillary service utilization, and other level-of-activity projections that are the basis for the revenue and expense estimates. Relevant statistics are utilized to construct *drivers* (defined activities) that cause variable budgeted costs to change in response to actual changes in the volume attributed to the driver. As the patient days for a specific program decrease, so should the costs associated with that program, including the relevant costs in nursing, ancillary departments, and support services. For some specific department-level costs, the patient days would be a driver. Within radiology, for example, the drivers would be the actual volume of each individual procedure. Changes in the volume of a specific procedure would change the requirements for the variable costs associated with the procedure and, therefore, the resource usage expectations, or budget, for the department.

The **cash budget** is a projection of cash balances at the end of each month throughout the budget year. This projection is based on operating cash receipts and disbursements, receipt or payment of loan principal, and capital expenditures. Because the cash budget compares the projected balances to established standards for desired cash balances, it provides management with a tool for projecting temporary monetary excesses that can be invested or shortfalls that must be covered. The cash budget combines information from the revenue and expense budget and the capital expenditures budget and, by doing so, often tests how well the two have been coordinated. In a sense, the cash budget tests the viability of the operating plan. The cash budget also focuses on the required stability of the budgeted and the actual net income. As volumes change, it must be management's objective to control related costs in response to the volume changes and maintain net income.

The **capital budget** is a plan that shows major capital expenditures for new equipment or facilities and for the replacement and/or modernization of existing equipment and facilities, along with the source of funding for the expenditures. To cover all resource requirements completely, the capital budget should include all capital expenditures (that is, all expenditures other than payment of loans that are not shown as an expense in the revenue and expense budget). This means, of course, that various levels of detail will appear in the capital budget. Large items will be shown and explained separately, whereas small items may be grouped and budgeted as a single amount for each month. Although the common budget period for the revenue and expense budget and the cash budget is one or two years, the capital budget usually covers a period of three to five years because of the lead time required to plan, fund, and acquire major asset items.

Because of their importance in budget preparation, statistics used to develop dollar amounts and statistics used to flex the expected expenditures (drivers) should be included in the budget package. They may be included in relevant explanations, as part of subschedules showing budget calculations, or as separate schedules supporting budget amounts.

The actual format for the various budget documents varies, depending on individual institutional requirements. The governing board may request specific schedules or analyses in reporting increases or decreases from prior-year projections or from prior-year actual amounts or in reporting compliance with regulations or debt requirements. For example, hospitals with significant debt typically show the calculation for debt service coverage and other ratios to demonstrate compliance with the debt covenants. The format of an individual budget may change to highlight a significant item. For example, few revenue and expense budgets included a separate line item for professional liability insurance prior to the large premium increases in the 1970s. Statewide uniform reporting requirements may demand a separate report from special responsibility center or account groupings in order to facilitate comparisons among institutions. This special report may be included in the budget package at the request of the governing board. As these examples suggest, the format of the operating budget should be adjusted to meet the needs of each institution. The budget process and the operating budget format vary for government hospitals, tax-exempt community hospitals, tax-exempt academic medical centers, large chains of investor-owned hospitals, or other types of health care facilities.

Types of Operating Budgets

The type of operating budget selected as well as the budget format depend on the organization's requirements. In general, there are eight or more types of operating budgets, among them responsibility and functional budgets, fixed and flexible budgets, program budgets, appropriation budgets, rolling budgets, and zero-based budgets.

Responsibility and Functional Budgets

A **responsibility budget** is one organized along established lines of management responsibility. Its basic unit is a cost center, a department, or a group of departments (an administrative unit) with a person responsible. Individual budgets prepared by each cost center manager are combined for a manager who is responsible for many cost centers. Similarly, budgets for an individual program may be combined with others for use by a manager who is responsible for a clinical service covering several programs. Organizing the budget along established lines of responsibility has the benefits of defining accountability for specific portions of the budget and controlling those portions to meet the budgeted levels of achievement. All budget packages, both department based and program based, should be organized and communicated along established lines of responsibility.

A **functional budget** is organized to identify such functional costs as nursing, housekeeping, and dietary services. One advantage of this type of budget is that service costs among hospitals can be compared. Advocates of this type of budget might include state rate-review agencies or other regulatory bodies. Because a functional budget does not relate to established lines of responsibility within an organization, it is not as useful for managing hospital costs and revenues as the responsibility budget is. The two types of budgets are not mutually exclusive, and both may be appropriate in the development and presentation of an annual budget. In those institutions where the organization of responsibility follows functional definitions, the two budgets may be the same.

Fixed and Flexible Budgets

A **fixed budget** assumes a single level of activity, and the entire budget is built around that level. For example, it can be assumed that the hospital has a complement of 238 beds that will not change during the budget period. Based on present occupancy and expected trends for each of the patient care areas, a utilization level of 74,708 patient days, or 86 percent occupancy, is assumed. The revenue and expense estimates will be based on the achievement of 74,708 patient days. The fixed budget would be an appropriate management tool if management could be reasonably confident that the volume and mix of patients will occur as expected. There was a period of years in the early and mid-1970s that this was true for many hospitals. But for most hospitals it is no longer true, and hospital managers must adjust resource usage to constantly changing volumes and mixes of inpatients and ambulatory patients. A fixed budget does not provide the support for monitoring and controlling resources in periods of change. For this reason, this edition will focus on the development and use of a flexible budget.

A **flexible budget** for the same hospital would reflect expected revenues and expenses at various levels of patient utilization. Because some costs are either fixed or semifixed (that is, they increase in a steplike fashion), the flexible budget usually estimates expenditures for ranges of activities. The flexible budget has the appearance of a series of fixed budgets at various occupancy levels. The flexible budget recognizes the difficulty of establishing a single optimum level of achievement and has the advantage of providing a tool for controlling costs at various levels. It may also have the effect of focusing on high-priority results, such as a desired operating margin.

When a hospital has a variable revenue and expense budget with an expected operating margin, it follows that the cash budget and the capital budget will focus on the expected margin, regardless of the possible range of variable revenue and expense. However, attaining such sophistication is a gradual process that is based on the successful development and implementation of fixed-level budgets.

The presentation of a flexible operating budget may appear similar to a fixed budget when it is finally packaged for presentation to the board of directors. The operating budget will reflect the anticipated results at an expected level of activity. The application of the flex concepts will be seen in the periodic reports that focus on the attainment of specific objectives, such as appropriate resource usage, and adjust the budgeted expenses to the actual activity on the basis of the specific activity indicators or drivers. The fixed budget becomes the adjusted expectation or desired result at the actual level of activity.

Program Budgets

The key to conceptualizing a program budget is a program matrix (figure 4-1). In a program matrix, program descriptions for all services appear on the horizontal axis and the resources (responsibility units) appear along the vertical axis. A program may be described as a set of activities related by a common goal or outcome and is often defined on the basis of principal diagnosis and/or operating procedures. For example, a perinatal program is a set of activities having as a goal the reduction of maternal and infant mortality and congenital disabilities through the provision of specialized services to a definite high-risk population. This set of activities requires the resources of a number of responsibility centers, such as nursing care, laboratory and other diagnostic services, dietary services, and housekeeping.

Because of limited space, the example of a matrix in figure 4-1 has only a few broadly defined inpatient services and programs on the horizontal axis and a few resources on the vertical axis. If all the significant programs were identified for inpatient, outpatient, educational, research, and other activities (such as the parking garage, professional building, and unrelated businesses), 100 or more items could be listed on the program axis. By relating the total resources of each responsibility unit to appropriate programs, the hospital can account for all revenue and costs of the units based on the support each provides to the various programs. Programs may be viewed as the product line of the physician–hospital joint effort.

One valuable characteristic of the matrix is that the total of the resource lines equals budgeted costs for the responsibility units, and the sum of a program's costs equals the total budget of the program. In turn, the total program costs equal the total responsibility unit's (department) costs, and the total departmental expense budget is allocated among services or programs.

The program matrix is a powerful tool for making decisions regarding the allocation of resources among various programs. It provides a link between planning and budgeting. The fact that this powerful tool is seldom used in the decision-making process suggests a lack of familiarity with the concept more than it suggests the degree of difficulty involved in developing the matrix. Defining a service or program is not always an easy task because of the necessity of obtaining agreement regarding which diagnoses and/or surgical procedures should be grouped together. However, agreement will evolve as management becomes familiar with the concept.

Programs may be defined not only according to diagnoses and procedures but also in terms of individual physicians, practice groups, or medical specialty groups. In such a matrix, the horizontal axis would account for all physicians, either as individual practitioners or practice groups if the medical staff is small or by clinical organization if the medical staff is large. Another approach would be to list medical specialty groups, such as cardiovascular surgery, orthopedic surgery, and pediatrics. All patients of a

Figure 4-1. Matrix for Relating Programs to Operating Units

General Hospital Budget—1990

	Inpatient									Total
	Cardiology				Gynecology		Neuroscience			
	Surgery									
	Open Heart									
	Coronary Bypass	Other	Other	Medicine	Surgery	Medicine	Surgery	Medicine	*Continued* →	
Nursing Units:										
Medicine/surgery	(a)									
Obstetrics										
Pediatrics		(a)								
Psychiatry										
ICU										
CCU										
Neonatal intermediate										
Neonatal intensive										
Nursery										
Ancillary Services:										
Operating Room: (b)										
½ to 1 hour										
to 2 hours										
to 3 hours										
to 4 hours										
More than 4 hours										
With heart pump										
Other										
Total Operating Room										
Labor and Delivery										
Anesthesia										
Post-anesthesia recovery										
Blood bank										
Laboratory										
Continued ↓										

(a) Units entered in the matrix could be recorded in terms of revenue, statistics, or cost.

(b) Operating room services are identified as an example of the charge structure that underlies the totals on each line. In the operating room the charge structure could, of course, be more specific than the example.

single physician would be listed in a single column along with all the patients of other physicians in the group. There would be no crossover of a physician's patients among programs as there is when diagnostic and/or procedure criteria are used for defining programs. This kind of matrix is easy to construct and is a satisfactory tool for short-term planning. It is also a good tool for improving communication among all members of the health care team.

Whereas the development of the matrix may have been extremely difficult several years ago, it is becoming easier as a result of more sophisticated cost-accounting systems and an emphasis on relating diagnostic information to patient bills for rate-review agencies and third-party reimbursement. When the hospital's programs can be defined by using diagnosis codes, the allocation of revenue and department costs can be based on an analysis of patient bills and the cost accounting for each procedure. In the absence of a cost-accounting capability, one can use the cost-to-charge ratios commonly used for calculating third-party costs to allocate department costs to procedures. Thus, the possibility of preparing such a matrix as a regular step in the budget process should be seriously considered.

Appropriation Budgets

Appropriation budgets are usually found in governmental organizations that depend on an outside source of funds, such as a tax authority or legislative appropriation. A single level of expenditures is assumed for a single level of activity. During the course of the review process, an outside agency reviews the budget line by line, approves or modifies the amounts budgeted for each line, and authorizes a specific expense amount. Each line item in the budget then becomes a maximum, and those responsible for carrying out the planned activities must obtain supplemental appropriations from the granting agency before exceeding the approved expenditure maximums. The use of a maximum often results in the tendency to spend the full amount appropriated.

Rolling Budgets

A **rolling budget**, also called a continuous budget, is one that is updated periodically during the budget period in preparation for the next budget cycle, which may be shorter or longer than a standard operating budget cycle. For example, a rolling budget for a 12-month period is reviewed and revised every quarter. The past quarter becomes history, and a new quarter is added to the projection to keep it moving ahead, or rolling, for the next 12 months. This type of budget is typically used for projecting cash availability. Receipt of a daily cash report and a cash forecast for the remainder of the week does not permit much time to react to significant change. Therefore, a cash projection for a three-month period may be requested and then updated every month.

Zero-Based Budgets

In a **zero-based budget**, senior management annually reevaluates all activities to decide whether they should be eliminated or funded. Appropriate funding levels are determined by priorities, the activities are ranked by top-level management, and projects are approved or disapproved according to the overall availability of funds.

Just as the program matrix helps to allocate resources among programs, zero-based budgeting concepts help to determine levels of resource requirements within a service or program and, therefore, determine optimum expenditure levels for each responsibility center. Largely because of the difficulty of segregating costs by service or program, managers currently budget incrementally. That is to say, some costs are added to, or subtracted from, the budget on the basis of the addition or deletion of specific services or programs (such as a new diagnostic service). However, most costs are increased by overall factors such as salary increases and by the impact of inflation on the cost of supplies without regard to services or programs; levels of input are not related to defined levels of output. As a result, each responsibility center concentrates on the justification for new costs rather than on normal increases in existing costs.

When zero-based budgeting concepts are followed, each responsibility center or department manager is required to justify the entire unit budget each year as if all of its activities were totally new. This is somewhat easier when a department's activities are spread across a program matrix. Department resource usage can be linked to programs of various priority and resource requirements. Once the concepts are adopted, management properly oriented, and the appropriate documentation and review procedures instituted, management is much better able to evaluate the levels of effort required to meet an operational objective as well as alternatives for achieving the same objective.

Zero-based concepts do not have to be applied to every responsibility center or department. They can be applied to some functional areas, such as travel and repairs, and to the staffing of some centers without a great amount of effort. In general, the concepts should be applied whenever possible. Unfortunately, the term zero-based budgeting brings to mind complicated forms, excessive documentation, and endless review. It does not have to be that way. Once the various activities of a department have been identified, the application of zero-based concepts should be a natural and relatively easy next step.

Chapter 5

Department Resource Management

Hospital managers have come to recognize the vital links that exist among effective and efficient resource management, economic viability, and the need for resource information for measuring results. A fully developed department resource management tool provides the department manager with the capabilities to do the following:

- Compare the department's actual expenditures by account to budget on a periodic basis
- Measure the department's labor productivity and monitor the productivity of individual labor categories in the department
- Develop individual procedure-level costs with identified labor standards for each procedure
- Relate the individual procedure volumes to changes in the caseload for particular types of patients

These capabilities are recognizable in the examples of department-level resource information shown in figure 5-1. The full strength of these tools is attained when the department manager is able to compare the actual to budgeted or expected results for each of the cost types listed and receive current variance or exception information on a regular basis.

In this chapter, an overview of the first of the three essential components of resource management information is provided, that is, the concept and development of procedure-level information that forms the basis for department-level resource management. The following two chapters address patient-level and program-level resource management and the aggregation of procedure cost and patient resource data to generate program-level costs (for example, pediatrics).

In order to manage a department effectively, a manager must have accurate, timely, and reliable information. He or she needs to have answers to the following questions in order to monitor the department's activities on a period-to-period basis:

- What procedures and what quantity of each procedure is the department producing?
- What are the time requirements for completing these procedures?
- What is the cost for producing these procedures?
- How do the actual labor, supply, and other costs compare to the expected costs for the volume of procedures provided?

Figure 5-1. Examples of Department-Level Costing Information

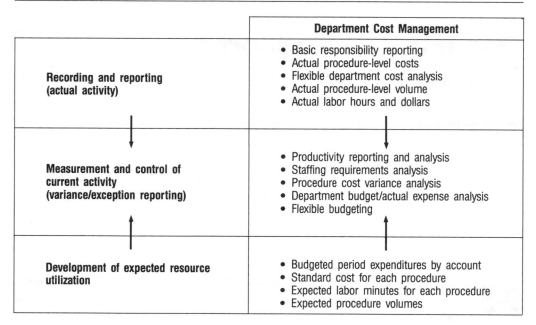

	Department Cost Management
Recording and reporting (actual activity)	• Basic responsibility reporting • Actual procedure-level costs • Flexible department cost analysis • Actual procedure-level volume • Actual labor hours and dollars
Measurement and control of current activity (variance/exception reporting)	• Productivity reporting and analysis • Staffing requirements analysis • Procedure cost variance analysis • Department budget/actual expense analysis • Flexible budgeting
Development of expected resource utilization	• Budgeted period expenditures by account • Standard cost for each procedure • Expected labor minutes for each procedure • Expected procedure volumes

This information can be obtained through the process of using procedure-level costing, integrating the individual procedure-level cost components into a resource management system that links the cost components to the actual and expected procedure volumes, and monitoring the cost components on a regular basis. It is a process that requires considerable effort, but the benefits are substantial. The objectives of procedure-level costing for department resource management fall into three categories: immediate, short-term, and long-term. The immediate objectives of procedure-level costing are the following:

- To develop more accurate procedure cost data
- To develop a deeper knowledge of procedure cost components (for example, time requirements per procedure)
- To develop the ability to compare budget versus actual costs at the procedure level
- To develop a methodology for ongoing maintenance

Short-term objectives are the following:

- To develop the ability to relay procedure cost data into a clinical/financial system for determining patient- and program-level costs
- To develop the ability to use fixed and variable procedure cost data for marginal costing and flexible budgeting
- To develop the ability to perform productivity studies
- To develop the ability to incorporate procedure cost data into actual and expected clinical treatment profiles

The long-term objective is to incorporate the procedure cost data into the program development, analysis, and monitoring that is an integral part of the strategic planning process.

Developing procedure-level costs, which focus on the department, precedes patient- and program-level costing because individual department services aggregated by patient are the foundation of all higher-order hospital cost analysis. Therefore, accurate determination of cost at the department and procedure levels is necessary if higher-order cost analyses are to be reliable.

Department resource management concepts can be developed in the relatively simple framework of the individual department, the basic management unit of responsibility. Focusing on the individual department minimizes the difficulty of defining interdepartmental relationships. Those relationships can be determined more easily once the resource management concepts have been developed in the departments.

Importance of Work Load Unit Measurement

Effective resource management at the department level requires attention to the department's *work load unit* – the unique output of each department. Department work load is measured in minutes per work load unit. Units can be defined by individual specific procedures, average procedure treatments, College of American Pathologists (CAP) units, Canadian work load units, adjusted patient days, or patient days per acuity level, to name a few examples. Care should be taken in the development of work load units for each department because similar work load units are needed to facilitate the comparison of results among hospitals. For example, it would confuse comparison if one hospital were to average one-day surgery patients with acute inpatient stay days and another were to account for them separately. Comparison is important because there are no universal standards for determining optimal performance.

As stated previously, department resource management should provide the department manager with accurate, timely, and reliable information regarding the cost of producing diagnostic and treatment procedures (as measured in work load units). This cost may be analyzed in terms of the actual labor cost compared to standard cost or the current period cost per work load unit compared to actual cost in previous time periods. To be effective, the department manager should be able to determine the different cost components included in the total cost for providing a single procedure. The cost related to technicians should be distinguished from supervisory cost, material cost, and support cost. The separate determination is required because cost related to technicians is affected differently by changes in output volume and mix than is supervisory cost, material cost, or support cost (allocated overhead). Technician cost is also managed differently from the other cost types.

There is a natural progression in the development of cost information. The information produced must include a determination of the cost per work load unit for managing the department resources and a determination of the total cost of each procedure in order to aggregate procedure costs by patient, by patient group, and by program.

For a large hospital with many departments, a complete list of department procedures might include several thousand items. Although this number of procedures may seem overwhelming, progress in developing useful resource information at higher levels ultimately depends on recognizing and controlling these procedure-level costs. Structuring resource management at the department level will facilitate a large number of simultaneous efforts, each involving hospital staff who are intimately familiar with the nature of their patient services and capable of providing useful assistance in developing cost information.

Basic Responsibility Reporting

Resource management tools must satisfy the department manager's need for reliable information at the department level that is produced on a timely basis and at an acceptable cost. For many hospitals the initial means for analyzing resource information will be the Receipts and Expenses Budget Report, as shown in figure 5-2. The hypothetical

Figure 5-2. Receipts and Expenses Budget Report for Period Ended May 31, 1990

Monthly Budget	Monthly Actual	Variance (Unfavorable)	Code	Description	Year-to-Date Budget	Year-to-Date Actual	Variance (Unfavorable)
$ 15,641	$ 6,737	$ 8,904	106	X-ray films	$ 61,946	$ 51,284	$ 10,662
22,287	28,310	(6,023)	126	X-ray contract media	88,266	189,542	(101,276)
2,620	410	2,210	164	Surgery-only instruments	10,375	7,896	2,479
4,358	0	4,358	165	Catheters	17,261	17,212	49
5,699	8,739	(3,040)	199	Other patient supplies	22,567	30,709	(8,142)
$ 50,605	$ 44,196	$ 6,409			$200,415	$ 296,643	$ (96,228)
$ 2,681	$ 4,398	$(1,717)	200	Printing, mileage, photocopying	$ 10,620	$ 14,596	$ (3,976)
$ 135	$ 295	$ (160)	400	Equipment, housekeeping	$ 535	$ 936	$ (401)
$ 53,421	$ 48,889	$ 4,532		Supplies and other expenses	$211,570	$ 312,175	$(100,605)
14,980	14,371	609	801	Radiologists	67,410	78,652	(11,242)
3,962	4,297	(335)	802	Joint clinical–medical	15,848	15,521	327
7,430	6,072	1,358	804	Residents	33,435	36,222	(2,787)
2,736	2,431	305	824	Charge nurses	12,330	11,278	1,052
4,068	6,784	(2,716)	825	Staff nurses	18,338	27,839	(9,501)
1,880	2,243	(363)	826	Enrolled nurses	8,478	9,682	(1,204)
69,462	65,245	4,217	848	X-ray technicians	286,068	297,636	(11,568)
27,364	26,150	1,214	849	Student X-ray technicians	109,456	104,892	4,564
$131,882	$127,593	$ 4,289			$551,363	$ 581,722	$ (30,359)
6,545	11,003	(4,458)	904	Orderlies	27,683	34,659	(6,976)
21,828	23,310	(1,482)	925	Clerical	98,226	103,504	(5,278)
$ 28,373	$ 34,313	$(5,940)			$125,909	$ 138,163	$ (12,254)
$160,255	$161,906	$(1,651)		Salaries and wages	$677,272	$ 719,885	$ (42,613)
$213,676	$210,795	$ 2,881		Department Totals	$888,842	$1,032,060	$(143,218)

example is for the radiology department at General Hospital. This department report depicts summary period results by expense code and expense grouping for the following items:

- Current month's budget and actual expense and budget variances (actual expenses minus budget)
- Year-to-date budget and actual expense and year-to-date budget variances

This report format, which highlights variances, can assist the department manager in effectively monitoring the department's expenses. The account descriptions classify the expenditures in functional groupings that are the foundation for procedure costing and that provide the detail for productivity monitoring. Although it is not shown in the example, the general ledger support also includes statistics. In addition to the actual month's salaries and wages of staff nurses, for example, the department manager should have ready access to the related paid hours broken down into regular, overtime, holiday, vacation, and sick time, together with the dollars related to each category.

In this first step, it is important that the hospital has a department and account structure so that departments are identified by the appropriate management unit and so that the appropriate accounts are established to adequately describe the costs within each department. That means the accounts contain the costs related to the service provided by the department, and the dollar amounts are supported by the appropriate statistics.

Although most hospitals have the ability to prepare such a period report, many hospitals do not have their account structure broken down into such detail by department. When it appears that the hospital's department/account structure is inadequate or too cumbersome, it should be corrected to ensure that the department resource management tool will be effective.

Procedure-Level Costs

Productivity analyses and procedure-level costs are directly related through the need to develop labor standards for each department-level patient procedure. Because of the relationship between labor standards and procedure costs, the two are often developed simultaneously. This section will discuss the costing process and then illustrate how the cost information and the labor components form the basis for department resource variance/exception reporting. The short digression from the process of budgeting to the process of costing is worthwhile because the procedure-level cost components are essential for the development of a sound flexible budget as well as for the development of patient-level and program-level resource management tools.

The objective of procedure costing is to use procedure-level labor standards, department and hospital statistical data, and budgeted hospital costs to determine the budgeted full cost of providing each individual hospital procedure. The format for the costing of procedures is shown in figure 5-3. This figure is for the radiology department at General Hospital and was produced on a microcomputer software package developed by KPMG Peat Marwick. Similar reports may be prepared using the costing software of several different vendors. This report depicts procedure unit costs by the following:

- Total variable and fixed costs per procedure
- Cost components of variable and fixed costs (labor, supplies, and so forth)
- Total unit costs

This sample format should be used to determine both budget cost per procedure (using budget department costs and expected volume for each procedure) and actual procedure costs using historical actual results for a recent period. Comparison of budget to actual costs and cost factors is needed to help evaluate the reasonableness of the assumptions used in developing the budgeted procedure costs.

The steps for performing the costing of individual procedures follow a logical order. The steps are not complicated, but because of the volume of procedures and the amount of data required, the process is time-consuming and involves the participation of many hospital personnel.

In planning and performing the costing process, the following important guidelines must be considered:

- The process should not be overly complicated. The calculation must be replicated or updated on a regular basis with only a portion of the effort required for the initial costing.
- Department management and staff must be involved in the costing. They know the procedures and are best qualified to identify the labor, supply, and other requirements. Because the cost requirements will be used to monitor department activity, department managers and staff should be comfortable with the factors included in the costing.
- Every procedure should be costed. Those 10 to 20 percent of the procedures that account for most (80 to 90 percent) of the resource usage will receive special attention in the process. The other procedures may receive less attention, but they should all be separately identified in the costing so that they can be reflected in the patient-level costs.
- All department and support (overhead) costs should be allocated to individual procedures. Noncontrollable, allocated costs can be separately identified by department managers because of the use of separate, detailed cost components. The total of budget procedure costs for a given period should tie to the total direct department costs and allocated costs for that same period. Costs such as those related to the president's office should be allocated to the appropriate

Figure 5-3. General Hospital's Summary of Average Costs by Procedure for the Diagnostic Radiology Department

Cost Center: Diagnostic Radiology
Cost Center Code: 6050

Procedure Code	Procedure Description	Total Adjusted Volume	Direct Labor Variable	Direct Labor Fixed	Direct Material Variable	Other Direct Fixed	Other Direct Variable
7102	Chest, 2 views	24,881	$ 6.65	$2.73	$ 2.02	$0.65	$0.00
7567	Body section	1,117	74.85	2.73	16.19	0.65	0.00
7331	Abdomen, multiple	4,711	13.72	2.73	2.67	0.65	0.00
7340	IVP tomograph	1,967	57.97	2.73	4.16	0.65	0.00
7301	Hip, complete	3,857	7.79	2.73	1.92	0.65	0.00
7220	Pelvis, AP only	2,332	7.02	2.73	1.18	0.65	0.00
7103	Chest, 4 views	2,892	13.37	2.73	2.67	0.65	0.00
7323	Foot, complete	2,540	12.16	2.73	1.09	0.65	0.00
7060	Skull, complete	924	16.74	2.73	1.83	0.65	0.00
7289	Hand, 1 film	2,692	5.79	2.73	0.71	0.65	0.00
7101	Chest, single	11,419	4.94	2.73	1.18	0.65	0.00
7557	Bone survey	129	19.88	2.73	4.54	0.65	0.00
7206	Spine, cervical	2,652	13.19	2.73	1.83	0.65	0.00
7566	Mammograph, bilateral	3,936	16.71	2.73	1.83	0.65	0.00
7215	Spine, lumbo-sacral	5,348	10.32	2.73	2.76	0.65	0.00
	All other diagnostic radiology	7,882	17.35	2.73	3.11	0.65	0.00
		79,279	$11.68	$2.73	$2.25	$0.65	$0.00

departments and included in the cost of the departments' procedures. They are a cost of the organization and a part of providing those procedures.
- The costs should be relatively accurate. They are used to monitor department activity and to develop patient-level costs and service-level costs.

As a result of completing the procedure costing steps, the hospital managers will have the following:
- Individual, accurate procedure costs for all major hospital procedures
- A methodology for calculating costs on an ongoing basis
- Computer software and hardware support on a microcomputer, a minicomputer, or a mainframe for updating the calculations on a regular, ongoing basis
- A manual that explains the costing in each department and identifies the individual procedure costs
- A data file in the hospital board's clinical/financial data base that contains the procedure costs and that will provide the basic cost elements for calculating patient costs and program-level costs

As a result of completing procedure-level costing, each department manager will have the tool needed to monitor and control department resources. The data will have been gathered, input to the central computer, and the initial reports prepared. The department personnel will be fully trained in the process and able to update the information on an ongoing basis. Each department manager will have the tools to do the following on an ongoing basis:
- Compare the department's monthly actual costs by account on a period basis
- Compare the department's actual work load units (volumes) to budget on a periodic basis
- Measure the department's labor efficiency
- Develop individual procedure-level costs

Figure 5-3. (Continued)

Physician Patient Care Variance	Physician Other Fixed	Subtotal Cost Center Expenses	Capital Fixed	Overhead Fixed	Overhead Variable	Total Expenses Fixed	Total Expenses Variable	Total Expenses Total
$5.17	$0.79	$ 18.01	$0.35	$10.59	$0.36	$15.11	$ 14.19	$ 29.30
23.50	0.79	118.72	5.59	69.80	0.36	79.56	114.90	194.47
7.99	0.79	28.55	0.39	16.79	0.36	21.35	24.73	46.09
23.50	0.79	89.81	1.92	52.80	0.36	58.90	85.99	144.89
5.64	0.79	19.53	0.23	11.48	0.36	15.89	15.72	31.61
4.23	0.79	16.60	0.21	9.76	0.36	14.15	12.78	26.93
6.58	0.79	26.80	0.75	15.76	0.36	20.69	22.98	43.67
4.23	0.79	21.65	0.38	12.73	0.36	17.28	17.83	35.11
8.93	0.79	31.67	0.98	18.62	0.36	23.78	27.86	51.63
3.76	0.79	14.44	0.17	8.49	0.36	12.83	10.62	23.45
3.76	0.79	14.05	0.26	8.26	0.36	12.70	10.23	22.93
20.68	0.79	49.27	0.64	28.97	0.36	33.79	45.45	79.24
5.64	0.79	24.83	0.40	14.60	0.36	19.18	21.01	40.19
13.63	0.79	36.35	1.05	21.37	0.36	26.60	32.53	59.13
9.87	0.79	27.13	0.30	15.95	0.36	20.42	23.31	43.73
9.81	0.79	34.43	2.85	$20.25	$0.36	$27.27	$ 30.62	$ 57.88
$7.10	$0.79	$25.21	$0.74					

The capability to relate the individual procedure volumes to changes in the caseload will result from the implementation of patient-level and program-level capabilities, as discussed in subsequent chapters of this text.

Variance and Exception Reporting

As stated earlier in this chapter, effective resource management at the department level requires attention to the work load unit—the unique output measure of each department. It is essential that the department managers have confidence in the defined work load units and that they have the ability to compare actual to budget volumes on a periodic basis.

It is possible that for certain hospital departments, the work load unit may have to be developed or revised in order to facilitate resource management. For example, a department may currently be recording the number of patients treated as its work load unit. Patients treated, however, may not be a true reflection of the department's output. This could be because the department treats many types of patients, or patient treatments vary considerably in resource usage. In this instance, the work load unit must be revised if the resource management tool is to be effective.

The emphasis in a productivity report is to compare actual hours paid to the required hours as calculated using actual procedure volume and the expected labor required for each procedure. The hours required are based on the time required to perform the actual volume of individual procedures (variable labor) plus the budgeted supervisory and clerical time, which does not vary with volume (fixed labor). The emphasis on variable labor will result in a renewed interest in the work load unit, which is the basis for calculating flexible hours.

The productivity information, which utilizes procedure-level labor data, can be monitored separately, or it can be incorporated into the flexible budget analysis. The flexible budget format analyzes the budget resources required for an actual level of activity. Labor requirements, which are a major resource in the flexible budget, are formulated on the basis of productivity expectations. Figure 5-4 shows a flexed budget report for the diagnostic radiology department at General Hospital. This particular report and those in figures 5-5 through 5-9 were produced on a clinical/financial soft-

Figure 5-4. Monthly Expense Variance by Expense Category Report

General Hospital Expense Variance by Expense Category
Report Period: July 1990 to June 1991
Cost Center: 6050—Diagnostic Radiology

Expense Category	Actual Expense	Flexed Expense	Budgeted Expense	Variances Rate/Efficiency (Flexed—Actual)	Volume (Budget—Flexed)	Total (Budget—Actual)
Labor (variable)	$258,950	$245,252	$252,147	$−13,698	$ 6,895	$−6,803
Labor (fixed)	42,450	37,500	37,500	−4,950	0	−4,950
Supplies (variable)	261,407	233,545	239,334	−27,862	5,789	−22,073
Purchased services (variable)	50,800	50,865	50,000	65	−865	−800
Professional fees (fixed)	105,000	100,000	100,000	−5,000	0	−5,000
Equipment depreciation (fixed)	150,525	170,000	170,000	19,475	0	19,475
Other (variable)	11,000	13,996	14,000	2,996	4	3,000
Facilities depreciation (fixed)	35,400	40,000	40,000	4,600	0	4,600
Other (fixed)	26,550	25,000	25,000	−1,550	0	−1,550
Total	$942,082	$916,158	$927,981	$−25,924	$11,823	$14,101

Note: A negative sign indicates an amount in excess of budget.

Figure 5-5. Monthly Labor Expense Variance Summary Report

General Hospital Labor Expense Variance Summary
Report Period: July 1990 to June 1991
Cost Center: 6050—Diagnostic Radiology

Staff Class	Description	Labor Expenses				Analysis of Labor Variance					
		Actual	Budgeted	Variance	Percent of Variance	Efficiency	Percent	Rate	Percent	Volume	Percent
CN III	Clinical nurse III	$ 77,450	$ 80,525	$ 3,076	3.82%	$ 2,083	67.74%	$ 209	6.80%	$ 783	25.46%
Senior tech	Senior technician	115,500	112,763	−2,737	−2.43%	−3,532	−129.06%	−2,028	−74.10%	2,823	103.14%
Tech	Technician	66,000	58,859	−7,141	−12.13%	−3,398	−47.58%	−7,032	−98.47%	3,289	46.06%
		$258,950	$252,147	$−6,802	−2.70%	$−4,847	−71.25%	$−8,851	−130.10%	$6,895	101.35%

Note: A negative sign indicates an amount in excess of budget.

Figure 5-6. Monthly Labor Rate Variance Analysis Report

General Hospital Labor Rate Variance Analysis
Report Period: July 1990 to June 1991
Cost Center: 6050—Diagnostic Radiology

		Wage Rates		Expense			
Staff Class	Description	Actual	Standard	Actual Hours	Actual Hours at Actual Wage Rate	Actual Hours at Standard Wage Rate	Labor Rate Variance
CN III	Clinical nurse III	$12.9950	$13.0300	5,960.00	$ 77,450	$ 77,659	$ 209
Senior tech	Senior technician	10.0260	9.8500	11,520.00	115,500	113,472	−2,028
Tech	Technician	10.1852	9.1000	6,480.00	66,000	58,968	−7,032
				23,960.00	$258,950	$250,099	$−8,851

Note: A negative sign indicates an amount in excess of budget.

ware package developed by and available from Health Care Microsystems, Inc. Similar reports can be produced from other commercially available software.

Each of the work load units (procedures) for the department is expressed in terms of minutes and represents the expected (or standard) time for completing a specific procedure. The use of an expected time, carefully developed with the people in the department who actually perform the procedure, enables department managers to analyze the resource input on the basis of what it *should be* for a given level of output.

The summary information in figure 5-4 shows that the department of diagnostic radiology incurred actual expenses of $942,082 for the period July 1990 through June 1991. In comparison to the original budget, the department incurred $14,101 more than budget. This report also shows that if the department expenses were compared to the budget adjusted for actual service volume, the overexpenditure would be $25,924—quite a different interpretation of the period activity in the department of diagnostic radiology.

To flex the budget, the original budget amount must be adjusted to reflect the actual volume, which was less than budget, and again to reflect the change from budget in the mix of the nuclear medicine procedures performed. Figure 5-4 shows the effect of the actual activity on those expense categories that are expected to vary or flex with changes in service activity volumes. The variable portions of labor, supplies, purchased services, and certain other categories of expense have been adjusted to reflect volume in the column labeled flexed expense. There is a volume variance for each of these categories. The fixed categories do not vary with changes in service volume. The amount in the flexed expense column is the same as in the original budget. It should also be noted that the categories in the Summary of Average Costs by Procedure (figure 5-3) are similar to the expense categories in figure 5-4. Had the two figures been prepared for the same institution, the categories would be basically the same with differences due only to the level of summarization on the cost summary.

The reports shown in figures 5-5 through 5-9 provide the detail needed to analyze the labor variance shown in figure 5-4 for variable labor. The summary report (figure 5-4) shows that labor costs for radiology technicians were more expensive than originally budgeted for the period, and after consideration of the decreased volume and the mix of services, the technicians were less productive than expected. The report in figure 5-8 shows the actual to budget variance in the volume and mix of service procedures.

The reports shown in figures 5-6 through 5-9 show the calculations for the labor rate, labor efficiency, and labor volume variances and illustrate the type of information

Figure 5-7. Monthly Labor Efficiency Variance Analysis Report

General Hospital Labor Efficiency Variance Analysis
Report Period: July 1990 to June 1991
Cost Center: 6050—Diagnostic Radiology

| Staff Class | Description | Standard Wage Rate | Hours | | Expense | | | |
			Actual	Earned	Actual Hours at Standard Wage Rate	Earned Hours at Standard Wage Rate	Labor Efficiency Variance	Efficiency Index
CN III	Clinical nurse III	$13.0300	5,960.00	6,119.89	$ 77,659	$ 79,742	$ 2,083	1.03
Senior tech	Senior technician	9.8500	11,520.00	11,161.43	113,472	109,940	−3,532	0.97
Tech	Technician	9.1000	6,480.00	6,106.61	58,968	55,570	−3,398	0.94
			23,960.00	23,387.93	$250,099	$245,252	$−4,847	0.98

Note: A negative sign indicates an amount in excess of budget.

Figure 5-8. Monthly Service Volume Variance Report

General Hospital Service Volume Variance
Report Period: July 1990 to June 1991
Cost Center: 6050—Diagnostic Radiology

Service Code	Service Description	Actual Volume	Budgeted Volume	Variance	Percent of Variance	Earned Hours
7510	Cerebral artery	1,383	1,400	17	1.21%	6,928.87
7520	Ankle, complete	1,721	1,700	−21	−1.24%	715.05
7530	Chest, single view	13,247	15,800	2,553	16.16%	5,744.22
7540	Chest, two views	7,377	7,300	−77	−1.05%	3,068.27
7550	Spine, cervical	658	600	−58	−9.67%	403.40
7560	Shoulder, complete	1,035	1,000	−35	−3.50%	428.40
7570	Tibia/fibula	1,633	1,500	−133	−8.87%	668.07
7580	Foot, complete	1,295	1,200	−95	−7.92%	531.19
7590	Paranasal sinuses	586	500	−86	−17.20%	471.03
7600	Pelvis	14,548	14,500	−48	−0.33%	2,350.06
7610	Urography w/tomograph	423	400	−23	−5.75%	454.58
7620	Urography	3,261	3,200	−61	−1.91%	1,624.80
		47,167	49,100	1,933	3.94%	23,387.94

Note: A negative sign indicates an amount in excess of budget.

a department manager needs to monitor department costs and productivity. The reports also highlight the importance of an accurate accounting of both budget and actual expenditures. If, for example, some of the radiology technician time that was actually spent to provide the procedures was incorrectly charged to another department, an incorrect conclusion regarding productivity might be drawn from these reports. An incorrect cost would have also been calculated for the service procedures provided by the department. A timely and accurate accounting of all resources used by the department is required to provide the department manager with the appropriate information for measuring and managing current department activity.

Conclusion

Referring back to figure 5-1, one can see that the steps outlined in this chapter would result in the development of decision support information for measuring and controlling current department activity. The system would be in place for comparing expected resource utilization with actual activity to determine, report, and analyze the following:
- The department's actual to budget expense variances, based on the actual level of activity
- Procedure cost variances
- Productivity measures

The basic data would also be available to analyze staffing requirements and actual to budget variances for specific department revenue or expense accounts.

Concerns about productivity and cost effectiveness are not new to hospital management, but the rapidly changing economics of health care, as described earlier in this manual, have served to increase their importance. The development of procedure-level costing and department resource management is the first step toward the creation of a complete resource management system that could improve a hospital's productivity and cost effectiveness.

Figure 5-9. Monthly Labor Volume Variance Analysis Report

General Hospital Labor Volume Variance Analysis
Report Period: July 1990 to June 1991
Cost Center: 6050—Diagnostic Radiology

| Staff Class | Description | Standard Wage Rate | Hours | | | Expense | | Labor Volume Variance |
			Earned	Budgeted	Earned Hours at Standard Wage Rate	Budgeted Hours at Standard Wage Rate	
CN III	Clinical nurse III	$13.0300	6,119.89	6,180.00	$ 79,742	$ 80,525	$ 783
Senior tech	Senior technician	9.8500	11,161.43	11,448.00	109,940	112,763	2,823
Tech	Technician	9.1000	6,106.61	6,468.00	55,570	58,859	3,289
			23,387.93	24,096.00	$245,252	$252,147	$6,895

Chapter 6

Patient Resource Monitoring

After procedure-level costs are developed for each patient service department, the next step is to link department procedures to the individual patients who received the services. By grouping patients (and the services they received) by contract, by clinical specialty, or by other program definition, managers and physicians can evaluate the resources utilized by that defined program.

Patient Resource-Tracking System

As departments perform procedures, the procedures must be assigned to individual patients. Department procedures are linked to individual patients through a patient resource-tracking system that collects current information from each department regarding the individual procedures received by each patient. The patient-specific data gathered include clinical data, demographic data, and the type and volume of procedures provided during an inpatient stay or an outpatient visit.

The patient resource-tracking system establishes a process for collecting procedure-level patient information and storing it in an automated form for merging with the clinical data currently collected for every inpatient. The tracking system provides the fundamental link that enables managers to identify specific procedures and procedure costs with individual patients. The billing system, which includes *detailed* charges for all patient services, provides the resource-tracking information for most hospitals. The key is to obtain the required level of detail through the charge detail and to accurately collect the data for costing and billing a patient stay.

The resource-tracking information is added to selected clinical and demographic data elements collected for each patient to form a large patient-specific data base. This data base combines the clinical, demographic, and utilization data from the billing file with the cost-per-procedure data and additional clinical data in order to analyze the resources utilized by a single patient.

Figure 6-1 illustrates the various uses of patient-level resource information for historical tracking, expectation development, and variance reporting. The charge capture and billing system tracks the procedures provided to each and every patient during the course of an inpatient stay or an ambulatory visit. Physicians can and will identify an expected treatment pattern for very specific groups of patients – groups

Figure 6-1. Examples of Patient-Level Resource Information

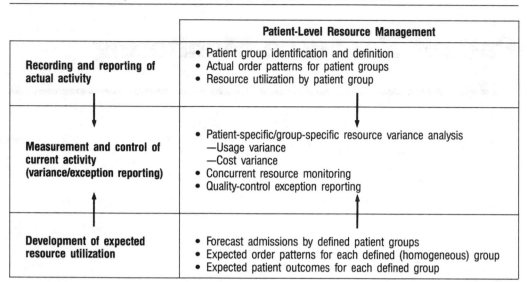

	Patient-Level Resource Management
Recording and reporting of actual activity	• Patient group identification and definition • Actual order patterns for patient groups • Resource utilization by patient group
Measurement and control of current activity (variance/exception reporting)	• Patient-specific/group-specific resource variance analysis —Usage variance —Cost variance • Concurrent resource monitoring • Quality-control exception reporting
Development of expected resource utilization	• Forecast admissions by defined patient groups • Expected order patterns for each defined (homogeneous) group • Expected patient outcomes for each defined group

who exhibit very similar problems when they are seen by the physician. By comparing the expected treatment pattern with the actual procedures ordered to diagnose and treat a patient, clinical managers can analyze the variance between the expected and the actual. Further, when the physicians have quantified the desired outcome for a specific patient group, given a defined course of treatment, the expected and the actual outcome can also be compared and analyzed.

Two basic efforts must be satisfactorily completed for these comparisons to be available. The first effort involves combining the financial data for each patient with the clinical data and demographic data in the patient resource data base. Financial data identify the individual procedures provided and billed to the patient. Clinical data identify information such as the patient's type of admission, primary and secondary diagnoses, and surgical interventions. Demographic data include such elements as the patient's age, sex, and home address.

Frequently, the accounts receivable bill file is the only source for the combined data. All of the data elements listed as examples in the preceding paragraph are included on a patient's bill. The effort involved is to improve the data on the bill file on the basis of more accurate and more complete data in other files. For example, the bill file may be the best source for a patient's address because, in most cases, a bill copy is sent to the patient's home. If the address is not correct, it will be returned. The bill file should also be the most complete electronic record of services provided to the patient. If it is not complete, a hospital department will not get credit for its efforts, and the hospital will not be paid for its services. If it is inaccurate, the patient, or more often the payer covering the patient, will question the services charged. The medical records file, however, is typically the best source for clinical information. To obtain the best data in the patient-tracking system, data will be collected from several different sources in order to improve and supplement the historical data in the billing files.

The second basic effort is to work with physicians to assign treated patients into meaningful homogeneous groups for analysis. Many of the common grouping methodologies developed for payment or other purposes do not identify clinically homogeneous groups of patients. Diagnosis-related groups (DRGs), for example, do not consider the stability of the patient at the time of admission. An unstable patient admitted to the hospital through the emergency department will typically require more services (more resources) than a patient classified in the same DRG who was admitted on an elective basis. The outcome expectations may be substantially different for the patient admitted through the emergency department. The effort involves working with the hospital physicians to define clinically homogeneous patient groups for the development of both practice profile (order pattern) and outcome expectations. One or more commercially available methodologies may satisfy the physician requirements.

Once sufficient and accurate data are available for analysis and the grouping methodology is in place, the treatment and outcome expectations can be developed and incorporated into the patient resource-tracking system. Variance analysis can then be accomplished at the patient level. This same data base is the source for marketing and other patient studies and is the basis for program budgeting and analysis.

Expected versus Actual Patient Resource Utilization

To develop a variance, there must be an expectation and there must be comparable actual results. In the case of patient-level resource management, the expectation is best expressed in terms of a clinical practice profile.

A *clinical practice profile* is a model of patient care that delineates the appropriate range in number and mix of services necessary for providing high-quality care to a very specifically defined (homogeneous) type of patient. This is a very important part of hospital resource management and a part that is of great interest to clinicians. Clinicians do not control the cost of a laboratory procedure, but they do control how often and on which occasions that procedure is ordered for all patients or any one patient. The effort to develop profiles is necessary for defining homogeneous patient groups for planning and resource management and for developing clinician expectations of resource usage for those defined patient groups. Because only a few hospitals have developed clinical practice profiles for resource management, the steps involved in developing a clinical practice profile are outlined below:

1. Select broad patient categories representing high-priority areas for the initial development of clinical profiles. A broad patient category can be represented by a DRG, a single diagnosis or group of diagnoses, or a condition requiring a specific type of treatment or procedure. The categories selected should represent high-volume/high-cost cases. Examples of broad patient categories include:
   - Coronary artery disease
   - Breast cancer
   - Diabetes
   - Normal delivery
   - Major joint procedures
2. Identify clinically homogeneous groups within each broad patient category. The most reliable way to determine whether a group of patients is clinically homogeneous is consensus among clinicians that patients are treated in a similar manner because of similar patient characteristics (for example, age, sex, disease severity) or the presence or absence of certain clinical criteria or events.
3. Delineate the appropriate number (in the context of a range) and mix of tests and procedures for each clinically homogeneous patient group. Once the clinically homogeneous groups are determined, clinicians can outline a model of expected resource utilization based on high-quality, cost-effective care. Using

historical information available in the resource management data base, the expected treatment plan derived from the clinical profile can be compared against actual treatment.

Figure 6-2 is an example of a clinical practice profile, and figure 6-3 is an example of a clinical practice profile variance report. The clinical practice profile in figure 6-2 provides the following information:

- Description of the homogeneous group using data found in the resource management data base
- Mandatory orders/treatments (procedures) and optional orders/treatments (frequently, contraindicated orders/treatments are also specified)
- Code and description for each procedure utilized
- Expected usage range (minimum, maximum, and average) for each procedure
- Cost range (minimum, maximum, and average) for each procedure
- Total expected costs

Because costs can be associated with each service, a clinical practice profile can be used to determine the expected costs of implementing the prescribed plan and the cost impact of underutilization or overutilization of services. Clinical practice profile variance reports (by department, physician, or patient) can document service and cost variances from the expected treatment.

Developing clinical profiles for new hospital programs provides valuable information about resource requirements. Linking clinical profiles with cost data is a critical step in developing budgets and new program requests. Clinical profiles provide the mechanisms to determining the department's needs on the basis of the projected number of cases, the number of procedures or tests per case, and the cost per procedure or test.

The resource management data can also be incorporated into the hospital's existing quality assurance programs. Each clinical profile represents a clinician-specified expectation of high-quality care for selected groups of homogeneous patients. In effect, the model represents a way to quantify quality by specifying the appropriate mix and number of patient care services. To enhance its use for quality management, each clinical practice profile could be expanded to include expected clinical outcomes. The critical indication of quality would be collected during the patient-tracking process and used for evaluating the actual outcome as compared to the expected outcome. The patient-level resource management tool, including expected outcomes, can be used to address a variety of quality-of-care activities:

- Quality assurance committee activities
- Peer reviews
- Utilization reviews
- Medical education

Improving the quality of clinical services through the use of clinical practice profiles will establish the hospital as a leader in quality management. Where applicable, clinical practice profiles provide the clinician with a means of demonstrating that the process of providing the appropriate resources to a patient to provide high-quality care is measurable and manageable. Having both process and outcome measures would greatly enhance any current quality assurance efforts.

Implementing a patient resource monitoring capability will give a hospital the management tool needed to monitor and control patient resources. Specifically, each hospital will gain the following benefits:

- Access to a sophisticated clinical/financial decision support system for patient-level information
- Information on the type of patients treated, the services used to provide care, the cost of those services, and the quality of care provided

Figure 6-2. Sample Clinical Practice Profile at General Hospital

Service: Medicine

Patient group: Acute myocardial infarction
ICD-9-CM Code 410–410.9

Subgroup: Acute admissions at time of infarction

Service Description	Procedure Code	Expected Volume per Patient			Expected Cost per Patient		
		Minimum	Maximum	Average	Minimum	Maximum	Average
Mandatory orders/ treatment:							
Daily nursing care	100	1	10	5	$265.19	$2,651.90	$1,325.95
Electrocardiogram (mobile)	C100	1	10	5	11.76	117.60	58.80
Chest X ray (simple)	M135	1	5	3	42.06	210.30	126.15
Complete blood count	85008						
	85570	1	2	1	21.86	43.72	21.86
Urea and electrolytes	82565	1	5	3	4.54	22.70	13.62
Erythrocyte sedimentation rate	85655	1	3	1	4.01	12.03	4.01
Cardiac enzymes	82550	2	5	3	4.98	12.45	7.47
Serum calcium	82320	1	2	1	3.30	6.60	3.00
Liver function tests	82400	1	2	1	4.00	8.00	4.00
Uric acid	84550	1	2	1	2.34	4.68	2.34
Glucose	84330M	1	3	2	2.44	7.32	4.88
				Subtotal	$366.48	$3,097.30	$1,572.08
Cardiology consultation							
Intravenous infusion							
Analgesia	Included in nursing cost						
Betablockers							
Vital signs							
Optional orders/ treatment:							
Coronary care unit	100	—	5	2	—	$1,847.20	$ 738.88
Lung perfusion scan	N504	—	1	—	—	160.18	—
Lung ventilation scan	N505	—	1	—	—	252.82	—
Echocardiogram	V115	—	1	—	—	81.54	—
Computed tomography	C305	—	1	1	—	263.73	263.73
Treadmill test	C105	—	1	1	—	111.44	111.44
Cardiac catheterization	C113	—	1	—	—	861.37	—
Catheter reporting	C119	—	1	—	—	105.62	—
Holter tape	1102	—	1	—	—	82.37	—
Swan–Ganz catheter	C117	—	1	—	—	480.44	480.44
Urinalysis	0628M	—	2	1	—	21.88	10.94
Cholesterol	82466	—	2	1	—	4.90	2.45
Hepatitis B agglutinin	86173	—	1	1	—	4.08	4.08
Prothrombin time	85730	—	5	3	—	22.90	13.74
Arterial blood gas	82884	—	3	1	—	18.57	6.19
Blood cultures	87512.0	—	3	—	—	28.74	—
Serum magnesium	83735	—	1	—	—	3.30	—
Drug levels	R200	—	—	—	—	39.80	—
Respiratory function test	RF101	—	1	—	—	67.45	—
Physiotherapy (15 min.)	P100	—	3	—	—	34.02	—
				Subtotal	$0.00	$4,492.35	$1,631.89
				Total	$366.48	$7,589.65	$3,203.97

Figure 6-3. Sample Clinical Practice Profile Variance Report at General Hospital

Fiscal Year 1991
DRG 106 Patients

Service Description	Total Number of Services	Expected per Patient		Actual Average Service per Patient	Average per Patient Outside Expected Range	
		Minimum Service	Maximum Service		Number Variance	Cost Variance ($)
Daily nursing care	335	9	15	11.03	0	0
Surgical intensive care	101	1	2	3.26	1.26	847.98
Swan–Ganz catheter	1	0	2	0	0	0
Arterial line	2	1	1	0	0	0
Bronchial treatment	297	0	9	11.42	2.42	63.90
Oxygen	108	1	2	3.26	1.26	55.58
Continuous ventilator	43	1	2	1	0	0
Medication nebulizer	18	0	9	0	0	0
Chest X ray	219	4	7	6.64	0	0
X-ray portable	162	1	2	4.91	2.91	98.91
CT head scan, plain	2	0	1	0	0	0

- The development of selected clinical practice profiles for planning and monitoring resource usage for specific patient groups
- An additional mechanism for monitoring quality of care through the clinical practice profiles

The hospital that completes the process outlined in figure 6-1 and throughout this chapter will have the decision support tool needed to compare expected with actual resource utilization on the patient level and to analyze the variances in terms of both cost and usage. With the clinical profiles for homogeneous patient groups, clinicians will have a solid methodology for enhancing current quality assurance efforts. The clinical practice profiles will also provide the basis for developing a tool for concurrent resource monitoring.

Chapter 7

Program Resource Management

Now that the hospital has determined the cost for each procedure and attached the individual procedures to specific patients, a third level of information is required to support a resource management system. This third level is program resource monitoring. During this process, the procedure cost and patient resource data are aggregated to generate program-level cost and resource utilization information. This information allows managers and clinicians to measure and monitor resource use by program. This effort links clinical and financial data at a macro or program level for planning and resource allocation.

Comparing Actual Utilization to Expected Utilization

The relationship between information describing expected results and actual activity is shown in figure 7-1. It is the same relationship that exists at the department level and the patient level. To manage effectively at the program level, the people responsible must have clearly developed program resource usage expectations, reports that show actual resource utilization for the same programs, and reports that compare actual to expected utilization. The variance reports should highlight the areas that require management action to obtain the expected results.

Why is this so important? Simply because most of the planning is done at a program level. The physician staff is organized on a program level. Most of the payment contracts are negotiated at the program level. Federal government payments are dictated at the program level.

Contracting provides an interesting example of the need for variance information at the program level, but it also provides an insight into a significant hospital management weakness. All too frequently when an opportunity arises for a hospital to contract for the care of a specific group of patients, the pricing decision is based on an estimate of what the market will bear without adequate knowledge of the cost of providing the necessary services. Later, after the contract is in place, there is not enough information to determine whether the pricing was appropriate. The actual cost of providing care to the contracted group remains unknown. With a majority of patients under one type of contract or another (Medicare, Medicaid, and Blue Cross are examples of larger contracts) and with no knowledge of the resources utilized to provide

Figure 7-1. Examples of Program Resource Information

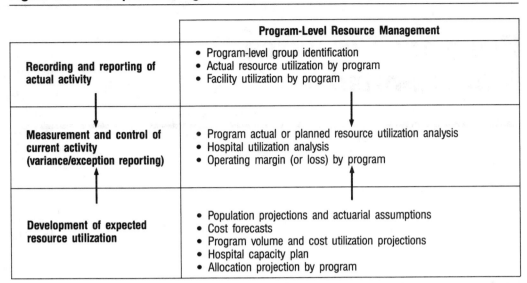

	Program-Level Resource Management
Recording and reporting of actual activity	• Program-level group identification • Actual resource utilization by program • Facility utilization by program
Measurement and control of current activity (variance/exception reporting)	• Program actual or planned resource utilization analysis • Hospital utilization analysis • Operating margin (or loss) by program
Development of expected resource utilization	• Population projections and actuarial assumptions • Cost forecasts • Program volume and cost utilization projections • Hospital capacity plan • Allocation projection by program

care to each of the contract groups, it should be hard to persuade purchasers, the board, or other hospital managers that available resources are being effectively managed.

Preparing Variance Data Using the Rollup Structure

The detailed data developed for managers at the department and patient levels are used to construct resource management information by program or contract group. The budget costs for individual procedures are summarized on the basis of expected order patterns for a specific group of patients as defined by diagnosis-related group (DRG), insurance code, age, or other patient-specific characteristics. The process sounds more difficult than it is. The data are available from the efforts to develop department-level and patient-level resource information. Historical data provide the basis for developing expectations.

As the program or contract continues, it is possible to compare the actual cost of providing the services with the expected cost. This comparison can be used to determine variances caused by variances in department-level costs, variances in physician order patterns, and variances in the volume and clinical classification of the contracted patients.

The reader should refer back to the matrix in figure 4-1, in which each of the columns in the matrix represents a program. The expected costs for each department to service the diagnostic and treatment needs of patients in the program are shown in individual program budgets. As stated in the diagram, the data in each cell (department/program intersect) could be stated in terms of revenue, cost, or statistics. The three-dimensional matrix accommodates any set of program definitions. The program description used to group patient data can be based on almost any program definition, such as clinical department, payer, DRG, or specific day surgery.

The program data accumulation using department-level and patient-level data in terms of various "rollup" structures further illustrates the concept. The hospital's patient-specific data in the resource utilization data base must be grouped according to specific criteria with a defined hierarchy in order to describe the resource utilization for specific programs. This hierarchy, or rollup structure, allows users to sum the detailed patient-level data and the more detailed department-level data so that the rollup structure mirrors the hospital's clinical structure, its services, and the related or homogeneous patient groups within each service.

Figure 7-2 illustrates a resource rollup from the procedure cost level to the highest level, which is the total cost of the hospital. At level 7 the individual costs, by component, are determined by specific department procedure. The procedure cost includes all the direct and overhead costs required to provide the procedure to any individual patient. Level 6 shows all the procedures provided to a patient during a specific stay in the hospital. A day of nursing care on a medical/surgical unit, a chest X ray, and a complete blood count (CBC) are just a few of many individual procedures, representing department costs, that might be provided during the course of a single inpatient hospital stay. Level 5 shows that the procedures relate to a specific patient who can be identified with an individual number and described by name. Level 4 recognizes the physician who was primarily responsible for the patient's treatment. Level 3 summarizes all of the procedures utilized for all of the patients under all of the physicians in the department of oncology. Level 2 further summarizes the clinical departments within the hospital management structure. The patients treated by all of the physicians reporting to the clinical managers represent the total resources used by the hospital during a given period of time (level 1).

As many rollup structures as desired can be created to characterize the operations of the hospital from different functional viewpoints. If the focus had been more on the payer, the rollup might have been structured as follows to reflect the total hospital cost identified by payer:

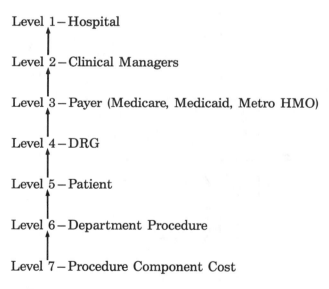

Level 1 – Hospital

Level 2 – Clinical Managers

Level 3 – Payer (Medicare, Medicaid, Metro HMO)

Level 4 – DRG

Level 5 – Patient

Level 6 – Department Procedure

Level 7 – Procedure Component Cost

The rollup structure can vary in terms of the grouping definition and the amount of detail. The number of levels can be expanded to provide more detail within each grouping, or it can be reduced to contain only summarized data at a few levels.

The rollup structure determines how cost, revenue, and utilization information are reported. Reports prepared using a defined program structure or rollup are based on a specific data set defined by the rollup. We have the ability, using this data set, to summarize the data for senior management review and then to quickly gain access to the appropriate detail for investigating and analyzing variances.

Figures 7-3, 7-4, and 7-5 illustrate the ability to view the same data in various levels of detail. Figure 7-3 is the summary matrix of the total resources utilized by

Figure 7-2. Example of a Rollup Structure

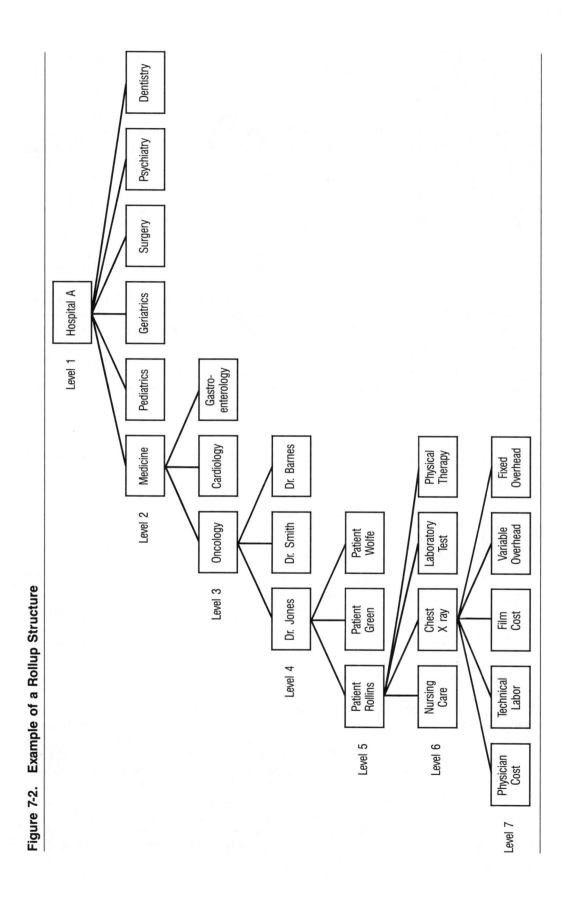

Figure 7-3. General Hospital's Analysis of Resource Utilization by Inpatient Service and Other Programs for Fiscal Year 1991

Department	Inpatient Care (by service) Medicine	Surgery	Pediatrics	Other[a]	Hospital Total
Nursing:					
1 West—Medical	$3,684,000	$	$	$	$ 3,684,000
1 East—Medical	3,097,000	—	—	—	3,097,000
2 West—Surgical	—	3,117,300	—	—	3,117,300
3 West—Surgical	—	3,400,700	—	—	3,400,700
4 East—Pediatric	—	—	688,200	—	688,200
5 East—Psychiatric	—	—	—	971,600	971,600
Hill Unit—Geriatric	—	—	—	627,500	627,500
ICU	—	—	—	3,845,700	3,845,700
CCU	—	—	—	810,000	810,000
Operating suite	21,700	3,398,900	3,600	379,800	3,804,000
Delivery suite	—	—	—	532,000	532,000
Radiology	428,200	1,335,100	164,900	1,445,800	3,374,000
Laboratory	883,500	1,981,400	169,200	2,503,900	5,538,000
Physiotherapy	84,400	168,300	36,000	289,300	578,000
Other	1,962,400	2,554,900	222,800	12,577,900	17,318,000
Totals	$10,161,200	$15,956,600	$1,284,700	$23,983,500	$51,386,000

[a]For purposes of this example, the inpatient cases relating to the other services, day cases, outpatient attendances by clinic, and community services by program have been grouped under Other.

Figure 7-4. General Hospital's Analysis of the Inpatient Cases within the Program: Orthopedics—Major Joint Program for Fiscal Year 1991

Department	Patients A	B	C	D	E	Other	Total
Nursing:							
1 West—Medical	$ —	$ 176	$ —	$ —	$ —	$ 824	$ 1,000
1 East—Medical	356	—	356	—	—	5,288	6,000
2 West—Surgical	6,502	2,288	3,244	5,632	176	147,158	165,000
3 West—Surgical	—	—	—	—	—	—	—
4 East—Pediatric	—	—	—	—	—	—	—
5 East—Psychiatric	—	—	—	—	—	—	—
Hill Unit—Geriatric	—	—	—	—	—	—	—
ICU	—	—	—	—	—	2,500	2,500
Operating suite	3,737	2,494	2,809	3,375	1,244	131,341	145,000
Delivery suite	—	—	—	—	—	—	—
Radiology	226	160	290	302	387	12,635	14,000
Laboratory	61	85	423	204	—	11,227	12,000
Physiotherapy/ occupational therapy	89	104	262	—	—	3,545	4,000
Central sterile supply	202	19	50	45	18	1,666	2,000
Emergency	—	—	—	—	68	432	500
Pharmacy	—	—	—	136	—	2,864	3,000
Totals	$11,173	$5,326	$7,434	$9,694	$1,893	$319,480	$355,000

Figure 7-5. General Hospital's Analysis of the Laboratory Resources Utilized by a Specific Patient during Fiscal Year 1991

Date of admission: 3-Mar-90
Date of discharge: 23-Mar-90
Primary diagnosis: 715.95
Secondary diagnosis: —
Surgical procedure: 815.9
Domicile: RR1, Sterling, IL 60010
Age: 86 years
Physician: R. Brown

Procedure	Number of Procedures	Cost per Procedure	Total Cost
Antibody titre	5	$18.31	$91.55
Additional cross match	8	8.52	68.16
Antibody screen	2	18.57	37.14
Cross match	2	12.45	24.90
ABO and RH group	2	8.99	17.98
Blood smear	5	4.64	23.20
Erythrocyte sedimentation rate	5	3.45	17.25
Coulter cycle	5	2.88	14.40
Other specific procedures	23	—	129.00
			$423.58

General Hospital during its 1991 fiscal year. The basic tool illustrated by the matrix enables the department manager to plan, budget, and manage resources on the basis of expected and actual volume changes in defined inpatient and outpatient programs. Similarly, a clinical manager can plan and manage with the knowledge of program resource requirements and the impact of program changes on the resources of any one department.

For example, a manager interested in the usage of laboratory resources might utilize the format in figure 7-3 to identify the overall distribution of laboratory resources by major clinical department. The next view might be a breakdown of surgery to identify the laboratory resources utilized by a new surgery program, such as orthopedics—major joints (figure 7-4). If the manager were using the data to forecast increased laboratory requirements based on an expansion of the new orthopedics—major joints program, he or she might be interested in the impact of an unusual case. It might be appropriate to break the data down further to the detail of the specific laboratory procedures for a high-utilization patient (figure 7-5) and discuss the requirements with a physician who is performing the surgery.

The technology to support this type of data manipulation is readily available from several vendors who support mainframe-based, minicomputer-based, or personal computer-based applications. Management's challenge is to develop the data at the department and the patient levels and to appropriately use the tremendous amount of data by turning it into useful information.

With this information, hospital managers and clinicians are able to do the following:

- Analyze historical demand for hospital resources by type of service (for example, medical, surgical, pediatrics, or any subset of these classifications) or by contract.
- Determine how to better allocate resources among services on the basis of expected patient requirements (this determination is the basis for the operating budget)

- Analyze the type of patients treated and the resources required for providing care by service or by contract, as compared to the expectation on which the allocation was based
- Assess the impact of change in service activity on the demand for tests and procedures by department
- Determine the need for capital by clinical service and by department

The combination of historical utilization information with service area demographic information enables managers to anticipate the demand for hospital resources and to focus available resources within the planning and budgeting process. It is this ability to utilize program information that provides the linkage between the planning and the budgeting process. Having determined the requirements by service, contract, and department, managers can compare actual to expected utilization. Any variance can be analyzed using the detailed assumptions on which the plan was constructed and the detailed actual utilization data in the data base. *The appropriate use of this department, patient, and program data is the basis for the type of budgets that hospital managers now need—program-based, flexible budgets that focus on the patients and their resource needs for high-quality diagnosis and treatment.*

Chapter 8

Budget Process

The process of putting together an operating budget extends from the review of the operating plan and the development of the budget package through the final approval by the governing board to the distribution of the approved department budgets to line managers. On the average, the process may take anywhere from 16 to 25 weeks. Putting the budget together is usually the responsibility of a budget director (or the person functioning in that capacity), who must be skilled and creative, patient but persistent, and knowledgeable about current operations. The emphasis is on coordination because the result of the process must be the institution's budget, not the budget director's budget.

All senior management and all clinical leadership should play responsible roles in the development of the budget. The chief executive officer is responsible for directing budget development. The entire budget package will have his or her signature on it when it is presented to the hospital's board of directors for approval.

Whether the effort must take the organizational form of a budget committee is a question each institution must answer. Typically, hospitals have a sufficient number of committees such that the budget effort can be organized within the responsibilities of an existing committee. Because of the involvement required of senior management, budget direction, resource allocation decision making, and progress monitoring should be a function of the most senior management committee, whatever it is called within the institution. Through this senior management group, individual duties will be delegated and progress will be regularly monitored.

As this book continually emphasizes, the budget is both a planning and a control tool. Its successful utilization requires the frequent monitoring of actual performance (as actual compares with expected performance) and the analysis of variance. Senior managers are responsible for monitoring ongoing programs for change, reduction, or elimination. The need for changes might be indicated by changes that occur in long-term objectives or changes that occur in the operating environment. Senior management is responsible for attaining budgeted results and for monitoring actual performance against budget on a daily, monthly, and yearly basis. The most senior committee is therefore the proper forum for directing and monitoring the development of the operating budget.

Medical staff management must also take an active and responsible role in budget development and performance monitoring. Without the direct participation of medical staff management, the budget committee would focus on expenditures based on "assumed" patient volumes. The appropriate participation of the clinical managers is for them to develop the program volumes (patient revenue) in the budget process and, as managers responsible for those volumes, to monitor the actual performance during the year. Clinicians should also participate in the development of patient requirements within a program. These patient requirements will further specify the volume expectations for each nursing, ancillary, and support department.

Prerequisites for Budgeting

The success of the budget process depends on the following elements:
- A set of well-defined policies, goals, and objectives to guide the resource allocation decisions
- An adequate description of current operations and the operating environment, including statistical data, economic trends, and demographic information for the area served by the hospital
- A defined budget period and established procedures for the development of budget documents
- A sound organizational structure that clearly identifies the department manager's and program manager's responsibilities and an accounting system that reflects the organizational structure and allows the revenue, costs, and relevant statistics to be accumulated and reported for each responsibility center and each program (in turn, each center can be grouped with other centers to reflect the full responsibility of each department manager, each clinical manager, and each member of senior management)
- Systems for the timely reporting of actual financial and statistical information for comparison with the budget and for analysis of variances (the reporting systems must be able to accumulate, compare, and summarize information for all responsibility centers and all defined programs)

Policies, Goals, and Objectives

The policies, goals, and objectives regarding strategic and operational planning were described in chapter 2. Also discussed in chapter 2 was the need for the planning documents to be responsive to the current and projected environment and for them to be approved by the governing board. The planning documents are an integral part of the budget process and are a constant reference for guiding decisions. However, because of the comprehensive scope of the documents, the budget manager may need to selectively summarize certain parts of the documents and include the summary statements in the appropriate sections of the budget manual. Furthermore, it may be more appropriate to include certain overall policies and selected objectives related to a specific responsibility center or program in that center's manual than to distribute the operating plans covering all centers and all programs to each line manager.

Budget development is a top–down process regarding what accomplishments are expected during the budget period (goal setting), a bottom–up response regarding the resources required, and a negotiation that results in the final allocation of resources needed to accomplish the hospital's objectives. To facilitate this process, overall guidelines such as the desired full-time equivalents (FTEs) per adjusted occupied bed, program priorities, and quality effectiveness criteria should be clearly communicated by senior managers at the very beginning of the process.

Description of Current Operations and Environment

In order to make resource allocation decisions during the budget period for such matters as salary levels, price increases for supplies, and current proposed new services, the budget committee and others involved in the budget process must have adequate data regarding hospital operations and the institutional environment. Many of these data are available from the environmental analysis performed as a part of the annual review and update of the hospital's strategic plan. The remainder of the data is available from current operating reports and projections made from these reports.

Budget Period

The defined budget period has typically been one year. However, it should be a two-year period with the specific allocations usually associated with a budget for the first year and less specific allocations for the second year. The budget period that most easily links to the planning process is two years because programs can seldom be planned and implemented in one year. Major adjustments to significant programs or changes in emphasis frequently take more than one year to plan and implement. A two-year period allows the program aspects to be budgeted generally in the second year and specifically in the current year. As the second year becomes the current year, the planned program volumes, revenues, and expenses can be reanalyzed and used as a basis for developing the current year's detailed budget. Programs can then be reanalyzed on a new two-year period. Any change in program priorities will be reflected in the current budget.

Each one-year period can be broken down into daily, weekly, or monthly segments for budget purposes. (It is helpful, for example, to get a daily revenue report showing actual versus budgeted revenue.) Established procedures enable the budget process to run smoothly if they are properly communicated and carefully followed.

Organizational Structure

The organizational structure reflects the delegation of authority and responsibility from the chief executive officer to individual clinical, program, and department managers. Each person's authority and responsibility must be clearly defined to facilitate a management system that involves each clinical, program, and department manager in budget development and then holds that manager accountable for actual performance as it is measured against the desired levels of achievement expressed in the budget.

Regardless of the formal organization, a successful budget process includes the participation of every person who has the potential to affect the operational outcome, such as the members of the medical staff. Once again, it is hard to understand how a hospital can estimate demand for its services without input from those most responsible. There is an old saying about trying to build a good house on a bad foundation. The same moral applies to demand studies and resource allocation decisions that are conducted without physician participation. As stated in a previous section, it must be senior management's objective to obtain physician participation in the budget *and* to obtain their agreement to be responsible for the actual results that are within their control. The medical staff must share in the responsibility for developing the budget and for attaining the budgeted results.

Reporting System

The reporting system is a basic tool for monitoring and controlling the progress of the hospital as it moves toward accomplishment of its long-term and short-term plans.

The information that management requires for control dictates the type, level of detail, and source of information collected and used in budget preparation. This required information also dictates the form in which the budget information appears in the final package. The reporting system that management uses for controlling the budget process should enable management to monitor levels of performance; to accumulate and compare actual results on a timely basis at the responsibility center, department, and program levels; to aggregate the comparative information for higher-level management reports; and to reflect the actual as compared with the budgeted results on a monthly or sometimes more frequent basis.

Work-Sheet Package

The package of work sheets distributed to department, clinical, and program managers at the beginning of the budget cycle usually includes the following:
- Cover memo
- Operating objectives for the department or program
- Detailed instructions with responsibilities indicated
- Calendar of deadline dates for the entire process
- Forms for completion
- Checklists for selected managers (optional)

The *cover memo*, which is signed by the chief executive officer, reminds all participants of the importance of the budget and management's support of the budget process. The memo may also be used to communicate certain underlying assumptions such as the inflation factors and the specific facilitywide goals or objectives established during the planning process.

The *operating objectives* are simply a reminder of the objectives developed during the planning process that are to be reflected in the budget for the department or program.

Instructions identify the scope and purpose of the budget program; outline the authority, duties, and responsibilities of specific managers or management groups; detail procedures for the preparation, review, revision, and approval of the budget; and provide samples of budget reports.

The *budget calendar* identifies the critical deadlines that must be met in order to complete the budget process on a timely basis. In setting up the time frames, the person responsible for preparing the calendar must take regulatory requirements into consideration. For example, the whole process may have to be completed in time for a review by a government agency before the beginning of the hospital's new fiscal year. The person preparing the calendar also needs to remember that those with budget responsibilities have other ongoing responsibilities. The budgeting process should begin early enough to give managers sufficient time to complete the budget steps as well as fulfill other management responsibilities. Typically, the reasonable period required for completing the budgeting process is closer to six months than to three months. For a medium-size or large-size hospital, three months will not be enough time to obtain the required management participation.

An example of a budget calendar for General Hospital for the year beginning January 1, 1992, is shown in figure 8-1. In the example, the time required between steps is shown as a range of working days needed to complete a particular task. Thus, this figure illustrates the timetable for a process that might be completed within 16 to 25 weeks. An actual budget calendar describes each step as well as the specific date of its expected completion. The actual completion date is also recorded.

Forms for completion, or work sheets, in the budget package are tailored to the information being requested and the person completing them. For example, the form

Figure 8-1. General Hospital's Timetable for 1992 Budget (December 31 Year End)

Activities[a]	Working Days	Expected Completion Date	Actual Completion Date
1. Senior management[b] [budget committee] meets to discuss: • Environmental analysis and operating plan • Economic assumptions • Operating policies, goals, and objectives • Budget timetable/responsibilities Additional meetings can be scheduled as required to complete the budget work schedule for each deadline.	—	_____	_____
2. Budget director distributes to department managers[c] the budget work-sheet package, which includes the relevant portions of the operating plan, operating goals, instructions, budget timetable, selected assumptions, work sheets for patient days and new and expanded programs, 1992 revenue and expense forms, and personnel budget (and possibly forms for reducing or eliminating current programs).	1–2	_____	_____
3. Budget director receives the projected statistics for patient days and ancillary utilization from administrative managers.[d] (The statistics forecast is prepared by department managers and medical staff.)	6–13	_____	_____
4. Budget committee meets to discuss: • Statistics forecast for patient days and ancillary utilization • Proposed rate increase parameters • Estimates of salary and wage increments	1–3	_____	_____
5. Department managers submit preliminary personnel budgets, expense and revenue budgets, and requests for new and upgraded positions (and deleted positions) to the appropriate administrative manager for review.	3–7	_____	_____
6. Department administrative managers submit new and expanded program requests to the appropriate administrative manager. They also review current programs against goals and objectives for possible increase, reduction, or elimination.	2–4	_____	_____
7. Each administrative manager submits the requests to add, expand, delete, or reduce programs to the budget director's office for consolidation.	4–9	_____	_____

(continued)

[a] Some of these activities may occur simultaneously.

[b] The membership of the budget committee should be indicated on the calendar, and any other appropriate individuals who should attend any or all meetings should be listed.

[c] Department managers may also mean cost center managers.

[d] Administrative manager may also mean director, unit manager, associate vice-president, or vice-president. Administrative managers are responsible for several departments and report to the hospital's senior managers.

Figure 8-1.   (Continued)

Activities[a]	Working Days	Expected Completion Date	Actual Completion Date
8. Proposed personnel budget requests, expense budgets, and revenue budgets are returned to the budget director by the appropriate administrative manager for consolidation into the hospital's overall budget.	1–1	_____	_____
9. Budget director submits a summary of new and expanded programs, new and upgraded positions, and programs proposed for reduction or elimination to senior management for review.	4–5	_____	_____
10. Budget committee meets to discuss proposals for new and expanded programs, new and upgraded positions, and reduced or eliminated programs.	2–5	_____	_____
11. Budget committee submits ranking for new and expanded programs and comments on programs to be reduced or eliminated.	5–10	_____	_____
12. Budget director distributes a summary of the 1992 budget, using the approved statistical budget that reflects reduced and eliminated programs but excludes new programs, salary increments, and new and upgraded positions.	0–3	_____	_____
13. Budget committee meets to approve the salary increment schedules to be utilized in the 1992 personnel budget.	2–2	_____	_____
14. Budget committee meets to review availability of funds to support inclusion of new and expanded programs in the 1992 budget.	0–5	_____	_____
15. Budget committee reviews the draft of the operating budget and discusses alternatives for resolving the net income deficiency (if applicable).	0–5	_____	_____
16. Budget committee approves final budget; by this date, any deficiencies should have been resolved.	5–10	_____	_____
17. Final budget is submitted to the governing board for initial review. (The budget should be in the mail 10 days before meeting.)	4–12	_____	_____
18. Budget receives final approval by the governing board.	10–22	_____	_____
19. Budget director distributes the approved 1992 budgets to the appropriate individuals in the hospital.	7–7	_____	_____

for submitting patient days should request that patient days be anticipated for each program for each month; it should show the actual patient days for each of the completed months of the current year and the projected patient days for the remaining months, as well as the actual patient days for each month of the preceding year. The breakdown of the patient days by program or service area reflects the organization of the hospital and the admitting patterns of physicians. For example, medicine, surgery, intensive care, cardiac care, obstetrics, pediatrics, psychiatry, and nursery are designated as separate service areas. It is desirable to further break down medicine and surgery days by floor or by nursing unit. (Samples of work sheets are shown in the following chapters.)

Checklists facilitate organizing and completing the budget process when a large number of persons is involved. Basically, the checklist is a detailed calendar with the steps to be completed and the dates of completion separately prepared for specific managers or groups of managers involved in the process. One approach is to prepare a detailed calendar showing each specific step for the entire process and then to circle those steps for which a particular manager is responsible.

Steps in the Budget Process

The flowchart in figure 8-2 shows the various steps in the process of developing the operating budget. On the average, the budget process takes from 16 to 25 weeks: 8 to 10 weeks for initial preparation; 3 to 4 weeks for consolidation; 4 to 12 weeks for review, adjustment, and approval; and 1 week for distribution. When the budget is prepared in a state that imposes rate review or other prospective review regulations, the process has to be initiated earlier in the year and/or compressed. Its output also needs to be adjusted to comply with the requirements of the appropriate agencies.

Following is a description of the steps outlined in figure 8-2. The number given to each activity corresponds to the numbers in the boxes on the flowchart.

Step 1. Long-Range Planning

The long-range goals and objectives are reviewed periodically by senior management (including clinical managers) and the governing board. *Before* each budget cycle, a new or updated operating plan is developed, as discussed in previous chapters. The goals and objectives in this plan are accepted as given and are not reviewed as an ongoing part of the budget process.

Step 2. Budget Format and Guidelines

At this point, the membership of the budget committee is reviewed, and members are appointed or reappointed. In most cases, the budget committee is made up of the hospital's senior managers in addition to the budget director and representatives of the medical staff. The committee has its first meeting or series of meetings of this budget cycle to review the economic analysis and the operating plan, decide the format of the final budget, establish preliminary assumptions with regard to rate increases and net income requirements, and establish the budget timetable.

Step 3. Volume Forecasts—Patient Days

Patient-day volume forecasts are prepared by the budget department on the basis of discussions with, and commitments from, clinical managers and in cooperation with nursing department managers, other department managers, individual admitting physicians, and planners. The patient-day forecasts are reviewed by senior management before inclusion in the budget. Admissions and patient days are forecast monthly for each major patient service area (medicine, surgery, intensive care, pediatrics, and so forth) and for specific programs within the major patient service areas. Changes in the expected length of stay and the impact of program changes on the patient acuity are also projected and analyzed at this time. In most instances, the forecasts are based on a historical trend analysis adjusted for expected program changes and for changes in medical staff, facility changes, and other anticipated events or conditions. Historical data and work sheets are supplied by the budget director. As a test of the reasonableness of the inpatient-day estimate, it should be possible for each clinical manager (for example, the chief of a specialty) to account for most (greater than 80 percent) of the expected patient days within his or her area of responsibility on an individual physician or practice-group basis.

Figure 8-2. Flowchart of Budgeting Process

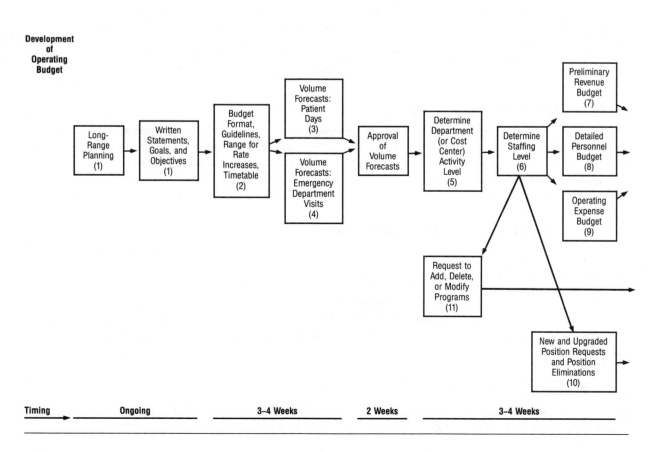

Furthermore, the patient-day projections should be analyzed by major payer group. How many projected admissions will be covered by Medicare? The days and admissions projected by payer should be reviewed for reasonableness considering projected payment terms, revenue and payer mix objectives, historical trends, and other factors.

Hospital managers with active emergency departments will also want to know how many and what type of admissions to expect through the emergency department. In line with the two-year budget concept, the forecasts should be specific for the current year and less specific, but still by program, for the second year.

Step 4. Volume Forecasts—Emergency Department Visits

Emergency department volume forecasts are the responsibility of ambulatory care department managers, in cooperation with physicians, planners, and the nursing service. Although this step refers to the emergency department, these forecasts should also

Figure 8-2. (Continued)

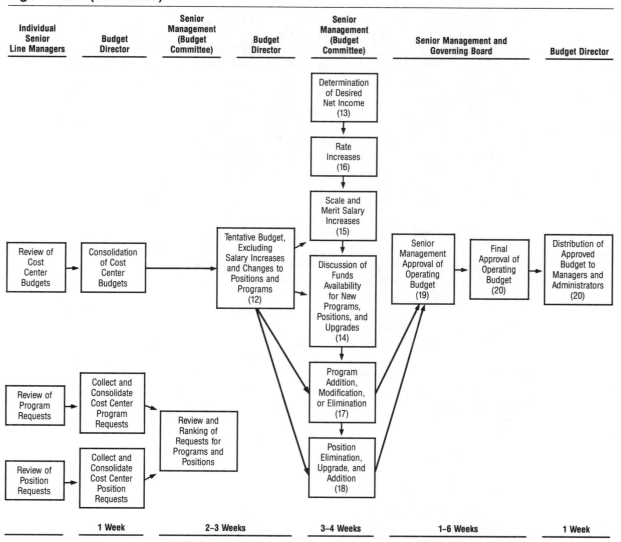

cover clinic visits if the hospital operates such a facility. As in the case of inpatient days, projections of visits are based on historical trends and other relevant factors.

Step 5. Department Activity Level

The overall projections of inpatient volume for patient care departments (for example, ancillaries) are based on the preceding year's ratio of procedures performed to patient days by program, that is, the number of tests performed based on the charges recorded. Departments receive daily, monthly, and end-of-year summaries of tests included in hospital revenue, and these data are the basis for making cost-center activity projections.

The historical volume trends and the relationship to an overall statistic such as patient days by program should be reexamined annually by those responsible for ordering the procedures—the physicians who practice within each program. Anticipated changes in the historical order pattern should be considered, as should any anticipated changes in order patterns resulting from new, available technology. Each department manager should seek the assistance of program managers, clinical managers, and individual physicians in order to anticipate volume changes resulting from the implementation of new programs or the reprioritization of existing programs.

Department activity levels should be projected for each procedure (at least each significant procedure). The reason for this detail is to incorporate the impact on staffing requirements of a change in the mix of procedures from, for example, the more mechanized tests requiring less manual input to the more exotic tests requiring substantially more staff time per test. Procedure-level detail enables the department manager to budget variable labor, supplies, and other expenses on the basis of the anticipated procedure volume and mix. This detail also enables the manager to recalculate and flex the staffing requirements on the basis of the actual procedures performed. The variable labor, supplies, and other departmental costs (calculated during the procedure costing study described in an earlier chapter), together with detailed volume projections, are needed to develop and utilize accurate flexible budgets.

Outpatient volume projections are based on historical emergency department visits, employee health care visits, and private outpatient statistics.

Support department (for example, housekeeping and laundry) projections are based on both inpatient and outpatient volume projections, with appropriate work-load measures (per day or per visit) used to estimate the required output (such as pounds of dry laundry) from each support department.

Projections for other support departments (for example, administration and finance) with no identifiable measure of output must be qualitative. These projections are often based on history and forecasted departmental changes. The much-preferred method is to use zero-based budgeting concepts and specific function analyses to project support requirements.

A general rule for all revenue-producing centers is that volume increases attributable to new tests or new programs can be projected only if the tests have been approved for that center or the program has been specifically identified in the operating plan. It is necessary to separately identify new procedures and new programs in order to compare volumes between years.

Step 6. Staffing Levels

Full-time equivalents (FTEs) are projected by job class, grade, and shift. The projections should be based on work-load requirements determined by using procedure-level projections for each department and work-load measures for each procedure (productivity measures). The projections should be reconciled to the preceding year's budget and should consider the approved additional positions and/or deletions during the budget period. The hospital should have a special process for approving changes in budgeted positions during the year. Each manager should have a method or process for changing staffing on the basis of the work-load requirements (a flexible budget control). The budget process should also include an evaluation of each department's current staffing levels based on the work-load or productivity ratios.

Step 7. Preliminary Revenue Budget

Projections of inpatient revenue for basic daily care are based on the projected volumes (patient days) for each cost center at the full price. Projections of nonpatient revenues (for example, parking garage, rents, and so forth) are based on activity forecasts and projected revenue growth.

Projections of gross ancillary revenues may use the following guidelines:

(a) Test volume projections are based on actual activity during the current year adjusted for known or anticipated changes resulting from patient mix, new procedures, or new programs. The volume projections should be based on a program model such as the matrix model discussed in chapter 3. Department managers must be provided with information on anticipated changes in patient mix or programs before being asked to estimate the budget year's activity. Each ancillary department volume should be based on the estimated requirements of expected program volumes.

(b) The price per test for each patient type is split into professional and technical components when appropriate. Department managers should use the price of their tests as reflected in the master price list, which is updated whenever rate increases are approved.

(c) Revenue by department (inpatient or outpatient) equals (a) multiplied by (b).

After the revenue budget is reviewed by the responsible senior manager, it is forwarded to the budget director. At this stage, revenue includes anticipated intensity changes in ancillary utilization (changes in historical physician order patterns). The budget committee reviews the assumptions used for the projection of ancillary services to ensure that all known or anticipated changes, before rate increases, have been considered.

The rate increases typically relate to a smaller and smaller group of patients whose insurance plan or self-payment covers the full fee. For most patients, the next step in the revenue budget is to calculate the net income on the basis of the contract terms and expected patient cases under each contract.

Net revenue is the amount that hospital managers really expect patients or their third-party payers to pay for services. It represents the discounted price. Net revenue is calculated on the basis of existing and anticipated contracts and contract terms. The analysis for the Medicare contract, for example, would include a projection of the inpatient cases covered by Medicare, grouped into DRGs and multiplied by each projected DRG rate. It would also include the numerous adjustments and calculations for exempt services. An analysis of the difference between projected total revenue from a payer and projected net revenue is the discount for that payer. Total revenue, net revenue, and the level of discounts for each major payer should be subjected to tests of reasonableness based on historical trends, anticipated program changes, hospital payer or revenue mix objectives, and other known factors.

Step 8. Detailed Personnel Budget

In preparing the personnel budget, department or responsibility center managers match the preceding year's personnel budget to the current payroll file; compare position descriptions, job class, salary, and number of authorized positions; and explain any discrepancies. Discrepancies usually result from positions transferred between cost centers or changes in job descriptions made during the year. At this time, senior managers should also review how well each department manager was able to flex the department staffing in relation to the patient work load. Did each department manager use available personnel efficiently?

The salaries in the personnel budget are based on current salary levels. If the hospital has a merit review program, it needs to consider the following when calculating individual salaries:

- If no review is scheduled between the present and the end of the current year, the current salary base should be used as the salary base for determining budget salaries and wages.
- If a review is scheduled, a new salary that would be in effect at the end of the current year should be estimated and used as the salary base for the budget year.
- If a position has a permanent shift differential, the differential should already be included in the base salary.
- Physicians' on-call premiums and nursing shift differentials are not included in base salary computations. They should be calculated and added separately to the department budget.
- Union increments effective between the present and the end of the current year should be included in the budgeted base wages for union employees.
- A proposed vacancy allowance should be calculated for individual nursing departments in order to project the dollar impact of unfilled positions. A separate vacancy allowance should be projected for each major department and in total for all other departments.

The corrected position control document for the current year and the personnel budget for each department should be submitted to the budget director only after they have been reviewed by the responsible senior manager.

Step 9. Operating Expense Budget

Salaries and wage projections are based on the current detailed personnel budget and adjusted for positions approved during the year. Overtime projections are based on projected overtime hours for each department or responsibility center. Supply expense projections are based on past experience and standards for individual patient services, and they are adjusted for expected volume increases/decreases related to anticipated program changes and price-increase (inflation) assumptions that are made at the beginning of the budget process.

Step 10. New and Upgraded Position Requests and Proposed Position Eliminations

New positions and requests for upgraded positions are usually based on increased work load, increased responsibilities, or new programs. Reductions in specific programs or eliminations of positions may be based on an overall review of existing programs in terms of their contribution to long-term goals and objectives or on a review of potential productivity increases resulting from new technology or improved techniques. The requests should be specific regarding the desired changes and the impact of the changes on expense and revenue. Before review and ranking by the budget committee, these requests should be reviewed by appropriate individual senior managers and consolidated by the budget director. The budget committee should also review the current and proposed method of staffing and payment to ensure that the individual departments develop and maintain the flexibility to adjust staffing on the basis of patient requirements.

Step 11. Requests to Add, Delete, or Modify Programs

Whenever a need for additional resources is determined, a request is submitted to the budget committee for review, approval, and inclusion in the budget. Additional resources that require approval include new and upgraded position requests and projects that cost $5,000 (or some other established amount) or more. Deletion or modification of any program that may have a significant effect on hospital operations should be similarly analyzed. The request should include the following information:

- Resources description and cost as well as the timing of the expenditure
- Indication of need with specific reference to the applicable programs in the operating plan
- Detailed description of new positions required
- Estimate of other direct and indirect expenses
- List of expected benefits of program (for example, cost savings, improved effectiveness, or improved department efficiency)
- Statement of capital requirements
- Statement of space requirements
- Description of expected impact on other cost centers
- Statement of the source of the necessary funds
- Approval of senior line managers

Forms used for requesting new programs include all of the preceding items in a simple format. Frequently, these forms become too elaborate, making them difficult to complete and difficult to review. Documentation is necessary not only for the approval process but also as a basis for evaluating the results of the program during the budget year and following years.

Before requests are submitted to the budget committee for review and ranking, the appropriate senior manager carefully reviews the requests from his or her responsibility centers and then submits those approved to the budget director for presentation to the budget committee. The requests for program addition, deletion, or modification are then reviewed and assigned priorities by members of the budget committee.

Evaluation of existing programs is difficult, but it must take place at this time in the process. Frequently, funds can be made available for a new program with a high priority only by eliminating or modifying a current program with a lower priority and redirecting the resources.

Step 12. Tentative Budget

The tentative budget includes the following projections:

- Revenue consists of inpatient service revenue, ancillary revenue, outpatient revenue, other income, and unrestricted gifts. Inpatient service revenue is budgeted patient days by type of service multiplied by the current average daily charge for nursing services. Ancillary revenue is the projected ancillary utilization by responsibility center multiplied by current rates. Outpatient revenue is the charge for clinic services, day surgery, and other ambulatory patient services. Ancillary revenue should be separately identified as inpatient or outpatient, if possible. Other income (for example, cafeteria and rents) is based on departmental projections. Nonoperating revenues are projected in line with historical trends. Unrestricted gifts are projected with input from the development office.

- Operating expense is an accumulation of cost center forecasts for each account. These are summarized in the categories of salaries and supplies. The budget director reviews overtime and other controllable expenses on a department-by-department basis to test for reasonableness.
- Free care is based on projections submitted by the finance department and reviewed using the economic assumptions in the operating plan. Free care identifies the subsidy of care for those unable to pay and includes an estimate for bad debts for those able but unwilling to pay.
- Contractual allowances are discounts offered to various third-party contract payers. These discounts are calculated on the basis of the terms of the contract, projected hospital utilization by patients covered by the contract, and current pricing. In most hospitals, Medicare is the largest contract payer. The discount shown in the budget is the difference between the listed prices for services to patients covered by a contract and the projected payment based on contract terms for those services.
- Vacancy allowance for all budgeted positions is based on a historical percentage of vacancies in relation to budgeted gross salaries and wages. The vacancy allowance is shown in the budget as an offset against the salary and wages expense.
- Depreciation is derived from lapsing schedules (or similar records) of existing assets and projected completion dates of projects in process.
- Interest expense reflects budgeted debt payment schedules and interest rates in effect for each type of financing. Interest income from invested funds is budgeted and shown separately in the tentative budget.
- Insurance calculations represent the cost of funding self-insurance or the projected premiums for specific types of insurance policies. The self-insurance portion is budgeted on the basis of actuarial estimates and funding requirements for the insurance period (which may or may not coincide with the budget year). The premiums for policies that are not self-insured are based on current quotations.

Step 13. Determination of Desired Net Income

The determination of desired net income is based on institutional operating margin requirements. These consist primarily of the need for working capital, plant and equipment capital, debt service coverage, and, in general terms, the maintenance of the value of the hospital's equity.

Step 14. Cash Availability

Cash availability is based on unrestricted funds available and the projected cash flow from operations. An overall projection of debt service and capital requirements can be used to determine reasonableness on an overall basis. The cash budget is a source of this required information.

Step 15. Scale and Merit Salary Increases

Scale and merit salary increases are suggested by the budget committee for each major employee category after consideration of the salary analysis submitted by the personnel director. Although a sum of funds is allocated to each department, it is expected that the increases will actually be determined and made on an employee-specific basis based on each employee's performance. Presumably, the amount allocated to each department will have a direct relationship to the performance of the department. In other words, the across-the-board increases so common in the past should be replaced by increases based on performance.

Step 16. Rate Increases

Rate increases for the average daily nursing charge are suggested by the budget committee. Any variance from the range originally established at the beginning of the budget process should be analyzed and discussed. Rate increases for ancillary procedures are suggested on a department-by-department basis and consider both program and payer utilization. Rate increases for individual procedures are determined after the budget has been balanced. Procedure charges should be based on the full cost of the individual procedure. In some instances, the charges are less than the full cost of a procedure. In these instances, other procedures may incur a higher charge to offset the deficit and balance the budget. This offset is commonly referred to as cross-subsidization. If cross-subsidization takes place within a department, it should occur as the result of a plan, not as a result of poor information or poor management.

In many instances, the actual rate increase is determined through a contract with a major payer. When establishing the rate increases for the budget year, senior managers must continually reconcile the increases to actual impact on the net revenue.

Step 17. Program Addition, Modification, or Elimination

Program additions, modifications, or deletions are approved by the budget committee for inclusion in the proposed budget after consideration of program priorities, availability of funds, and the level of additional expense the hospital can afford given proposed operating margin requirements.

Step 18. Position Elimination, Upgrade, and Addition

New and upgraded positions are determined in the same manner as new programs. Any decisions that result from this step will be reflected in the hospital's position control system as well as in the department and program budgets.

Step 19. Budget Committee Approval

Budget committee approval of the operating budget follows the committee's review of the first budget draft to determine that net income and projected increases in net revenue are within guidelines established at the beginning of the budget process. When the budget is not within these guidelines, expenses are reanalyzed on a departmental basis for reasonableness in relation to the reduced revenue or net income, with close attention paid to controllable costs. New programs, scale and merit salary increases, new positions, and existing programs are adjusted until a balanced budget is obtained. *Balanced* in this context means that net patient revenue plus other revenue minus all expenses results in the required net income.

At this point, the cash budget, the capital budget, and the projected balance sheet, which have been developed concurrently, are finalized and made a part of the full budget package. All elements of the package are then reviewed and balanced before final approval.

Step 20. Final Approval

Final approval of the operating budget begins after the budget has been approved by the budget committee. It is then submitted for approval to senior management, the appropriate state agency (if necessary), the executive committee or finance committee of the governing board, and finally to the full governing board. The final approved budget is distributed to the appropriate line managers. Numerous reports are provided to various levels of management during the year to assist them in managing ongoing operations.

Chapter 9

Net Income

To meet its total financial requirements, a health care institution must maintain a margin of net revenue in excess of total expenses (net income). This margin provides the necessary funds for working capital, plant and equipment capital, and for investor-owned institutions, an amount equivalent to the dividend requirements of its shareholders. The need for a sufficient net income is simply a recognition of the fact that health care institutions cannot survive in the long run if they operate at the break-even level, where only operating expenses are recovered and no additional funds are available for capital replacement and growth. Prudent managers maintain the financial stability of their institutions in order to fulfill their responsibility to the community they serve. During the past 5 to 10 years, hospital managers have increasingly used debt to replace assets and to add new assets. *However, debt is not a means of ensuring financial stability. Debt is no substitute for net income; it is a mortgage on future net income.* Many managers who found it easy to incur debt to replace assets are now finding it difficult to meet the debt payment requirements and at the same time replace assets and provide for growth.

Net income is as much a requirement for tax-exempt health care institutions as it is for investor-owned institutions. The difference in the amount required by these two different types of institutions is equal only to the portion of income applicable to dividends of investor-owned institutions.

Net income is the bottom line on the income statement. Nonoperating income is a part of net income and should be included in the budget. Some institutions depend on contributions or income from investments to generate sufficient net income. In essence, these sources of income are a reduction of the income to be generated from patients. In such cases, it is essential that the required contributions or investment income be included in the budget. As a rule, all sources of revenue as well as all expenses should be included in the budget.

A desired or required level of net income should be stated in the institution's operating plan and in longer-range financial forecasts. If it is not, the budget committee should establish the net income objective in the first few meetings of the current budget cycle. In either case, net income requirements should be included in the determination of revenue and expense, and the net income reflected in the preliminary revenue and expense budget should be in line with the net income objective. Before the preliminary revenue and expense budget is considered to be complete, net income requirements must again be analyzed to verify that the budgeted net income is adequate. At this point in the budget process, the cash budget and the capital budget should be nearing completion and should provide some of the information necessary for evaluating the adequacy of the budgeted net income.

During the budget year, as actual revenue and expense are monitored in comparison to budget, the net income objectives should remain as a constant. Management must not allow overexpenditures or changing utilization to reduce net income. Rather, expenditures must be managed to maintain net income. At the end of the budget year, an ineffective manager might attempt to rationalize a net income lower than budget by citing changes in payer mix, utilization, and expenditure requirements. An effective manager would explain how expenses were managed as payer mix and utilization changed in order to protect and maintain the budgeted net income. *Because they realize their responsibility to the community and to future generations, effective managers make sure that the institution's financial requirements are met.*

Working Capital and Capital

Working capital and capital were defined in the 1981 AHA publication *Operating Margin for Health Care Institutions* (Chicago: American Hospital Association, 1981, pp. 1–2) as follows:

> Working capital is defined as current assets less current liabilities. The Policy on Financial Requirements of Health Care Institutions and Services recognizes this accounting definition, but focuses on the institution's "having sufficient cash to meet current fiscal obligations as they become due." The minimum working capital requirements of a health care institution for any budget year consist of the additional funds needed (1) to cover expenses during the time lag between the provision of services and the collection of charges, (2) to maintain or build inventories in advance, (3) to provide for increasing insurance premiums on prepaid insurance, and (4) to provide cash reserves for contingencies. . . .
>
> Capital requirements are the portion of projected capital needs for which funds must be set aside each year. Funds for projected capital needs should be prospectively accumulated in order to prevent the need for unreasonably large amounts of debt to fund large capital undertakings or to defer a necessary capital project because the required funds are not available. Capital requirements are determined through the capital budget in accordance with anticipated needs as reflected in long-range planning, institutional policy, and management decisions. Capital requirements will generally include amounts for the following circumstances:
> - Anticipated major construction, renovations, repairs, and proposed acquisitions resulting from expansion or new technology
> - Replacement of current plant and equipment that reflects changes in prices and new technology

If the budgeting process outlined in this book is followed, a projected statement of changes in financial position will be developed. The model operating budget includes such a statement, which shows how the funds developed from net income and other sources are applied to working capital and plant and equipment capital. The statement for a hypothetical institution, General Hospital, reformulated slightly for this analysis in figure 9-1, shows that net income and depreciation provide funds equal to $2,068,000. In addition, changes in the working capital transactions for other accounts receivable; accounts payable; and salaries, wages, and other accruals provide

Figure 9-1. Analysis of Net Income Requirements

General Hospital
Analysis of Net Income Requirements—1992 Budget

Funds will be provided by:		
Net income		$ 996,000
Add: depreciation that does not require outlay of funds		1,072,000
Funds available from operations and nonoperating income		$2,068,000
Working capital transactions		
Decrease in other accounts receivable	$ 30,000	
Increase in accounts payable	200,000	
Increase in salaries, wages, and other accruals	220,000	450,000
Total funds available		$2,518,000
Funds will be utilized for:		
Capital		
Payment of long-term debt		$ 215,000
Purchase of property and equipment		1,016,000
Increase in funds designated for future expansion		590,000
Working capital transactions		
Increase in cash and investments	$200,000	
Increase in patient services receivable	421,000	
Increase in other current assets	76,000	697,000
Total funds used		$2,518,000

another $450,000 for a total of $2,518,000. These funds will be used for capital requirements, that is, to pay debts, purchase equipment, provide for future expansion, and meet working capital requirements related to increases in cash and investments (the reserve for contingencies), in patient services receivables, and in other current assets. If all of the assumptions made by General Hospital are correct, the funds available from net income will be used as projected in the analysis.

Is it enough? Did General Hospital meet the requirements as outlined in the *Operating Margin for Health Care Institutions*? If the assumptions were correct, the net income would cover the working capital requirements, including the $200,000 increase in cash and investments to be reserved for contingencies (figure 9-1). Whether a $200,000 increase in cash and investments is sufficient for an institution of this size is a management decision.

Did General Hospital meet its capital requirements by providing for "anticipated major construction, renovations, repairs, and proposed acquisitions resulting from expansion or new technology" and for the "replacement of current plant and equipment that reflects changes in prices and new technology"? Without knowing about any anticipated major capital projects, one can evaluate the amount available to replace current assets by applying the generally accepted accounting principles for price-level changes. Although the hospital provided $1,072,000 through depreciation of property and equipment, it should have provided through depreciation and net income, approximately $1,962,000 just to *replace* its current property and equipment, based on an analysis of price indexes for the years in which the various elements of property and equipment were purchased. Therefore, the hospital did not meet its financial requirements. If the hospital cannot meet its financial requirements by providing enough funds from operations to replace its property and equipment, it is simply consuming its capital and slowly destroying itself. Only an irresponsible management would allow this to occur.

Once the working capital and capital requirements have been determined, the excess or deficiency should be highlighted for the budget committee and the governing board. A statement on the excess or deficiency of funds required over funds available explains how the funds required were determined and the impact as well as the suggested corrective action.

In summary, the development of an operating margin or net income is accomplished through the budgeting process. The adequacy of the net income should be determined according to management's best judgment regarding future events and specific criteria, as discussed in this chapter.

Departmental Contributions

To help each line manager understand the need to contribute to the institution's net income, the institution may adopt a broad policy that in effect states that every revenue-producing department must contribute a certain percentage over and above its direct costs to cover revenue deductions, indirect costs, and other financial requirements. That is one approach. Another approach is to have a policy that indicates the desirable income from each department after both direct and indirect costs have been considered. The latter approach assumes the ability to perform a full cost analysis of budget data in the relatively short time available in this part of the budget process. In the current health care environment, this is a requirement and a reasonable expectation where a significant percentage of the hospital's services are covered by payers that pay the full charge.

Using the broad approach first, for example, the institution sets the contribution margin (gross revenue minus direct costs) at 58 percent for this budget. The 58 percent is calculated on the basis of total revenue deductions, indirect costs, and the net income requirements as outlined in this chapter. Because senior management and members of the governing board established the policy, they will want to know how well each department measures up to its goal. It is likely that some departments, such as the emergency department, will not be able to contribute 58 percent; therefore, other revenue-producing departments will have to contribute more than 58 percent in order to bring the overall contribution to that level.

The format in figure 9-2 can be used to communicate these relationships. Including such a schedule in the budget submitted to the governing board should be considered, along with an explanation of the contribution policy and the reasons for variances.

The problem with the contribution margin approach is the increasingly irrelevant hospital charge structure. In the first place, the charge structure of many hospitals has little relationship to the cost of providing services. That may be the case either because management ignored costs over the years or because a conscious effort was made to increase charges for those departments that were used most frequently by charge-paying patients.

As more and more payers contract for deep discounts and pricing becomes increasingly based on per case, per capita, or per diem rates, department charges become less meaningful. The disparity between total patient revenue (based on charges) and net revenue (the actual amount that the hospital expects the responsible party to pay) has grown in some hospitals to as much as a 50 percent discount. In other words, net patient revenue is approximately 50 percent of total patient revenue. At some point, a contribution analysis based on hospital charges loses its value to managers and

Figure 9-2.   Analysis of Departmental Contributions to Net Income

General Hospital
Analysis of Departmental Contribution for Budget Year 1992

Basic daily services:	Contributions (%):
Medicine	69
Surgery	68
Intensive care unit	37
Cardiac care unit	49
Pediatrics	66
Obstetrics	69
Nursery	62
Ancillary services:[a]	
Operating room	55
Recovery room	51
Delivery room	55
Central supply	67
Intravenous therapy	45
Emergency department	49
Anesthesiology	66
Day surgery	35
Laboratory	43
Blood bank	49
Electrocardiology	43
Cardiac catheterization laboratory	51
Radiology	58
Ultrasound	44
Electroencephalogram	43
Respiratory therapy	42
Physical therapy	46
Pharmacy	65
Nuclear medicine	64
CT scan	39
Overall	58%

[a]Includes inpatient and outpatient services.

heightens management's awareness of the disparity between the amount paid by those few payers that pay the full charge and average payers that receive a deep discount. The preferred approach to managing and communicating each department's contribution is to focus on actual cost (including support or overhead costs) and net revenue.

If the capability exists to perform the cost allocation for the determination of the allowances for third-party payers (described in chapter 8), the same information may be used to analyze the net contribution of each revenue-producing department after allowances and indirect costs. Such an analysis might follow the format shown in figure 9-3, which basically is a statement of departmental profit and loss from patient services. The adequacy of this income or the total net income is the subject of another analysis. This schedule shows how much each department contributed to the net income from patient services. Columns to the right of the 1992 net contribution figures may be added for comparable dollar amounts from 1991, unit-value revenue and expense analysis, cost-to-charge ratios, or payer-mix statistics. Figure 9-3 is an informative summary analysis, and consideration should be given to including it in the budget package along with a complete explanation of its relevance.

Figure 9-3. Calculation of Net Departmental Contribution for Budget Year 1992

General Hospital
Performance Analysis for Budget Year 1992

Service	Patient Revenue	Deduction from Revenue	Net Direct Expense	Indirect Expense	1992 Net Contribution
Basic daily services:					
Medicine	$ 3,255,072	$ 314,440	$1,021,966	$ 1,529,884	$388,782
Surgery	4,239,687	409,554	1,356,670	1,967,051	506,412
Intensive care unit	680,034	65,691	428,961	300,017	(114,635)
Cardiac care unit	715,742	69,141	367,871	348,372	(69,642)
Pediatrics	373,797	36,109	127,091	194,374	16,223
Obstetrics	681,543	65,837	211,278	361,217	43,211
Nursery	175,140	16,918	66,553	92,824	(1,155)
	$10,121,015	$ 977,690	$3,580,390	$ 4,793,739	$769,196
Ancillary services:[a]					
Operating room	$ 1,619,000	$ 156,395	$ 724,502	$ 705,723	$ 32,380
Recovery room	283,000	27,337	137,736	106,607	11,320
Delivery room	266,000	25,695	119,700	125,925	(5,320)
Central supply	1,109,000	107,130	365,176	527,974	108,720
Intravenous therapy	732,000	70,711	401,551	281,698	(21,960)
Emergency department	1,214,000	117,272	616,712	674,256	(194,240)
Anesthesiology	174,000	16,808	58,500	62,152	36,540
Day surgery	40,000	3,864	25,948	13,388	(3,200)
Laboratory	2,769,000	268,043	1,578,330	888,468	34,159
Blood bank	301,000	29,076	152,667	116,247	3,010
Electrocardiography	276,000	26,662	158,037	83,021	8,280
Cardiac catheterization laboratory	369,000	35,645	179,850	135,055	18,450
Radiology	1,215,000	117,369	510,300	550,881	36,450
Ultrasound	42,000	4,057	23,447	13,565	931
Electroencephalogram	53,000	5,120	30,321	18,089	(530)
Respiratory therapy	511,000	49,363	296,380	155,037	10,220
Physical therapy	289,000	27,917	157,116	121,307	(17,340)
Pharmacy	1,380,000	133,308	477,480	637,412	131,800
Nuclear medicine	143,000	13,814	52,181	56,985	20,020
CT scan	287,000	27,724	175,070	66,986	17,220
	$13,072,000	$1,263,310	$6,241,004	$ 5,340,776	$226,910
	$23,193,015	$2,241,000	$9,821,394	$10,134,515	$996,106

[a]Includes inpatient and outpatient services.

Chapter 10

Units of Service Forecast

As discussed in chapter 8, much of the budget development process requires the use of costing procedures and information on patient days or visits and ancillary procedures. Because the whole budget process may be stated in terms of dollars and statistics, both historical and projected, reliable statistics are as important as reliable cost data. Statistics are used to estimate the volume and scope of activity for budgeting and, of course, are an integral part of all federal and state reimbursement and rate-setting systems. Statistics are used to manage according to the budget and to flex the budgeted costs to actual volumes. In addition to having the statistics related to hospital operations, managers responsible for budget preparation need to have access to statistics on relevant environmental trends, economic factors, and demographic data related to the hospital's immediate service area. These data are important in projecting the health care needs of the community and in developing and analyzing proposed new services or programs to meet those projected needs. Written procedures in the budget package should describe the statistical data to be gathered, the method of accumulation, and the preferred methods of statistical projection preparation.

Steps in the Forecasting Process

Basically, the steps in gathering and forecasting units of service are these:
- Selection of the appropriate unit of measurement
- Accumulation and analysis of the historical data for at least the past three years
- Review of the relationships between program volume and ancillary utilization
- Verification of the relationships with program managers and clinical managers
- Preparation of preliminary forecasts based on historical program data
- Adjustment of the preliminary forecasts for anticipated program additions, deletions, or modifications and for other known or anticipated internal and external factors
- Verification of the forecast utilization with program managers and clinical managers
- Comparison and coordination of individual forecasts to develop an overall institutional plan
- Finalization of individual forecasts

The responsibility for gathering statistics and preparing the forecasts should be specifically assigned. The logical person for this job is the department manager. However, the direction for gathering the statistics should come from the budget committee. Some statistics are available from several sources and so can be compared for reasonableness before being used in the budget process. For example, radiological procedures recorded by the radiology department can be compared with billing records for the same procedures and an explanation obtained for any significant variances. Another example is the number of meals served, which relates closely to the number of patient days in acute service areas (other than intensive care and nursery).

The best method is to project department volumes on the basis of projected change in the volume and mix of patients through the use of concepts discussed in chapter 4 and methods discussed in chapter 5 and chapter 7. To develop these projections, the budget director along with clinical managers and program managers should analyze the hospital's current and historical experience. Together they should examine the relationships between program volume and ancillary utilization. These relationships should be examined by type of patient within a program or clinical service. The analysis should cover inpatients, day-surgery patients, and other outpatients. The objective of such an analysis is to develop a model for projecting utilization on the basis of the projected volume and mix of patients. Projections will take into consideration expected changes in the order pattern for particular types of patients, changes in the community's demand for services, changes in the technology available, changes in payers' expectations (as expressed through payment changes), and changes in the medical staff.

In most cases, it is the responsibility of the budget manager to gather relevant current and historical data, to coordinate the analysis by clinical and program managers, and to present the projections in a format for use by the line department manager for analysis and comment. As in the case of any projection, the data must be accompanied by information on assumptions, explanations, and other relevant comments if they are to be useful for the department manager.

Given the projection, it is each line manager's responsibility to comment on and revise the statistical forecasts for his or her department on the basis of known factors in addition to the program assumptions. These department statistics are important to each department manager because they will provide the foundations for expected labor, supply, and other cost requirements, they will be the basis for flexing the department budget during the year, and they will form the basis for establishing and monitoring efficiency expectations for the department. In all cases, it is the responsibility of the budget committee to review all statistics and approve them before they are used in the budget.

Given the importance of these statistics, the remainder of this chapter is directed toward those who are developing budget statistics for the first time. The chapter can also be used as a reference for those who are reevaluating their system for accumulating and analyzing budget statistics.

Some statistics, such as the number of medications dispensed or laboratory tests performed, are the product of ongoing operations and should be easily obtained from hospital records. Other statistics, such as the amount of engineering or building maintenance time utilized by each department or the pounds of laundry processed, require special studies or a change in data collection systems. Often, an analysis of historical trends adjusted for known changes in community requirements, hospital facilities, and other environmental factors provides a reasonable basis for budget estimates.

The level of sophistication in the gathering and use of statistics varies from hospital to hospital. The range of sophistication in the development of patient revenue statistics can vary from calculation of patient days multiplied by an anticipated per diem, to patient days for anticipated routine revenue and anticipated ancillary utilization by department, to anticipated routine and ancillary utilization by admission. The range can also vary by type of admission. Clearly, any manager utilizing the per diem method understands the difficulty of managing according to the budget and will want to move quickly to develop the ability to prepare projections based on expected utilization by type of admission.

There is a risk that too many statistics, conflicting statistics, or irrelevant statistics will be gathered. Time spent on analyzing useless statistics is, at best, time wasted. Throughout the budget process, decisions must be made concerning the usefulness of certain statistics in relation to the effort required to gather and analyze them and the value of the statistics in actually managing the hospital resources.

The budget director assists the line manager in making statistical projections in numerous ways. For example, the budget director may use any one of several different forecasting methods, such as an index method or a linear regression graphical approach. The budget director may also prepare these projections separately and then compare them to the projections prepared by the line managers as a test of reasonableness. Particular care must be taken not to become so dependent on a method of forecasting that the ability to determine the reasonableness of the result is lost. Results must be analyzed closely, and changes in current conditions must be examined and factored into the projections. Statistics change. A simple extension of current trends will not be appropriate in most instances. Changes such as the following would affect any projection based solely on historical utilization:

- The mix of patients may change and cause a change in the demand for services.
- New facility construction or renovation may add to, subtract from, or change the type of services available.
- New programs may add new services or change the availability of current services.
- Population changes over time may lead to new or changing demands (for example, an influx of young families may increase the demand for pediatric services).
- Changes in the medical staff may change demand for services.
- Changes in the diagnostic and treatment order pattern for any specific type of patient may change the demand for specific services.
- Changes in the financing of health care may affect available services.
- Changes in state and federal regulations may affect the availability of resources and specific services.
- Changes in the economy may affect the demand for, and the availability, of certain services.
- Changes in the services offered by other hospitals in the area may affect demand.

Enough data should be available to consider these possibilities in the analysis of variances for the current year and the development of a budget for the next year.

The following example illustrates the point. In order to perform an overall analysis of expenditures for a certain group of inpatient pharmacy items, the price and volume variances could be calculated. The actual price multiplied by the actual number of prescriptions compared with the budgeted price per prescription multiplied by the actual number of prescriptions yields a price variance. The actual number of prescriptions multiplied by the budgeted price per prescription compared with the budgeted number of prescriptions multiplied by the budgeted price produces a volume variance. As price and/or volume change, enough data should be available to explain the changes in terms of the possibilities listed in the preceding paragraphs.

Careful analysis of statistics is essential. The forms designed to accumulate statistics should be specific as to the statistics' nature and source. For example, a procedure is not always a procedure: it may be one of a package of procedures, with the package counted and billed as a single procedure, or it may be a quality control procedure run several times with different methods or equipment to verify accuracy (and not be captured using the charge structure). Definitions of the statistics are important, as are coordination and consistency in gathering statistics. A basic test for reasonableness is to determine consistency within the budget process by comparing changes in statistics to known environmental forces expressed in the strategic plan, new equipment in the capital budget, and previously approved programs.

Patient Day Statistics

Historical patient day statistics and budget projections should be classified in several different ways:
- By payer for estimating contractual allowances and uncollectible accounts
- By accommodation (single-bed room versus two-bed room) for estimating gross revenue
- By service, for determining gross revenue and net revenue by service (for example, general medicine, intensive care, or nursery), estimating ancillary services required (for example, operating room, catheterization laboratory, or radiology), estimating nurse staffing requirements (for example, intensive care, intensive care nursery, or pediatric specialties), and estimating capital requirements (for example, radiology equipment, blood bank supplies, infant warmers, and physical therapy equipment)

The statistics for payer breakdown are usually derived from an analysis of billing data. For monthly reporting, this may be shown in tabular form for the end of a given period or graphical form for the year to date to reflect trends.

Accumulation of patient day statistics is best done from census reports. The typical daily census report (or midnight census) is done by nursing station and is summarized by service. One format for such a report is shown in figure 10-1.

Having a correct bed complement statistic is important. An endless stream of questionnaires ranging from regulatory agency surveys to information updates for various association data bases comes to every hospital. Because it is difficult to monitor the hospital's responses to all questionnaires, the information commonly available on such standard reports as the daily census needs to be consistent and accurate. It is embarrassing when several different agencies have received different information from the hospital regarding bed complements and therefore have different occupancy

Figure 10-1. Sample Format for Daily Census Report

General Hospital
Daily Census Summary—Census at Midnight (September 12, 1991)

Service	Previous Census	Admissions	Discharges	Transfers	Current Census	Bed Complement	Occupancy (%)
Medical	74	10	14	2	72	76	94.7
Surgical	93	11	10	—	94	101	93.1
Intensive care unit	10	1	1	(2)	8	12	66.7
Cardiac care unit	9	—	—	—	9	12	75.0
Pediatrics	12	1	3	—	10	15	66.7
Obstetrics	13	3	1	—	15	22	68.2
Total	211	26	29	—	208	238	87.4
Nursery	6	2	1	—	7	11	63.6

percentages recorded for the institution. It is even more embarrassing when members of senior management cannot agree on the census or on patient day statistics because different results were obtained after gathering the statistics from different sources or at different times of day. Anything as basic as a census count should not be a matter of routine controversy.

This same census information should be summarized for each month of the year and for the year to date, and it should be included in the monthly financial statements as supplemental information. A sample format for the monthly/year-to-date summary is shown in figure 10-2. However, it might be more useful to separate the information into two reports, one showing statistics for the current month and the other showing statistics for the year to date. An alternative approach is to record patient days on one report and percent of occupancy on another. Similar reports may be prepared on the basis of admissions for the month and for the year to date or on the basis of the average number of beds occupied.

Estimates of Patient Days and Admissions

Monthly inpatient utilization is important for estimating cash flow and for analyzing and controlling on the basis of actual activity. Monthly utilization is also important for estimating personnel requirements. If monthly utilization is coordinated with full-time and part-time staff availability, vacation schedules, and estimated sick time, overtime requirements and/or agency staffing requirements can be anticipated.

Given the program analysis described in previous sections of this chapter, the two sample formats shown in figures 10-3 and 10-4 can be used for analyzing and reporting forecasted patient days by service and accommodation. The sample format for analyzing and reporting forecast patient days by service (figure 10-3) is most effective when the actual patient days for the prior months and years are recorded by the budget director and presented along with the program or service forecasts. The administrative and medical staff are then asked to complete only a patient day forecast for the budget year. The patient day forecast is based on the program forecast. The medical staff probably will take the opportunity to comment on the reasonableness of the patient days budgeted for the remainder of the current year, and their comments should be solicited. In fact, their comments should be solicited each and every month. However, if new information concerning the current year arises during the budget process, it should be acted on. A memorandum summarizing the budget assumptions that affect patient days should be distributed along with the schedule and the program analysis. This is a good way to test the budget assumptions and to communicate to the medical staff and the nursing staff such significant anticipated events as the completion dates for new construction, the timing and extent of anticipated renovation projects, and the addition, expansion, or contraction of any inpatient service.

An analysis similar in format to figure 10-3 should also be prepared to show forecasted admissions. It too should be analyzed and accepted by the medical staff and the nursing staff. The sample format for analyzing and forecasting facility utilization (figure 10-4) is a useful schedule for estimating revenue, especially when revenue is based on patient days and ancillary utilization by department or by type of admission. When there is not a substantial difference between the charge for a one-bed room and a two-bed (or multibed) room, the information required for budgeting revenue can be taken directly from the sample format for analyzing and forecasting patient days by service (figure 10-3).

As an alternative, the budget director may complete the budget projection for the coming year as well as record actual activity for the prior years and the projection

Figure 10-2. Sample Format for Monthly and Year-to-Date Census Summary

General Hospital
Comparative Statistics on Hospital Occupancy—September 1991

| Service | Bed Complement End of Month | Patient Days | | | | | | Percent of Occupancy | | | | | |
| | | September 1991 | | 1990 | Year to Date 1991 | | 1990 | September 1991 | | 1990 | Year to Date 1991 | | 1990 |
		Actual	Budget	Actual	Actual	Budget	Actual	Actual	Budget	Actual	Actual	Budget	Actual
Medical	76	2,164	2,143	2,168	19,772	19,793	19,731	94.9	94.0	95.1	95.3	95.4	95.1
Surgical	101	2,824	2,806	2,812	25,698	25,781	25,615	93.2	92.6	92.8	93.2	93.5	92.9
Intensive care unit	12	242	243	246	2,257	2,251	2,244	67.2	67.5	68.3	68.9	68.7	68.5
Cardiac care unit	12	270	257	256	2,391	2,369	2,270	75.0	71.4	71.1	73.0	72.3	69.3
Pediatrics	15	299	243	248	2,580	2,273	2,265	66.4	54.0	55.1	63.0	55.5	55.3
Obstetrics	22	451	446	457	4,336	4,144	4,132	68.3	67.5	69.2	72.2	69.0	68.8
Total	238	6,250	6,138	6,187	57,034	56,611	56,257	87.5	86.0	86.6	65.6	65.1	64.8
Nursery	11	210	205	203	1,928	1,892	1,877	63.6	62.1	61.5	64.2	63.0	62.5

for the current year. The appropriate administrative and medical staff can then review the projection for reasonableness on the basis of the projections of patient days by service in the program analysis and their individual expectations. The budget manager should not do so much work on the projections that the administrative and medical staff give the budget only a cursory review. If the result of the process became the "budget manager's budget," the budget would not be a useful tool for managing resources during the budget year. Regardless of who prepares the forecast, it is essential that the medical staff supports the forecast and that the month-to-month statistics are forecast to the best of their ability. The statistics will be the basis for forecasting nurse staffing requirements, monitoring physician activity, and determining the reasonableness of ancillary departments' monthly forecasts.

Forecasts of Physician Activity

In order for the budget to be an effective forecast, the individual members of the medical staff must agree to its reasonableness and be willing to have their performance measured against it on a monthly basis. To ensure the budget's usefulness as a test of reasonableness and a tool in developing the medical staff's accountability, several more steps are required at this point in the budget development process. The first step is to determine the admissions (and the patient days) for which the medical staff is accountable. Generally, the physicians should not be held accountable for admissions through the emergency department or through the clinics. If the hospital has an active emergency department and active clinics, admissions from those areas should be forecast and monitored separately. Similarly, if a substantial number of admissions are the result of a contract with a health maintenance organization or a similar managed care program, the accountability for admissions should be separately monitored. The other admissions (commercial insurance patients, Medicare patients, and others) are the result of patients' relationships with individual physicians and should be forecast and monitored by physicians (or physician groups).

Figure 10-5 is an example of how the forecast admissions might be analyzed. The service breakdown by clinical area relates to the clinical managers responsible for each service. The admission totals should be tied to the forecast of total admissions prepared in a format similar to figure 10-3. Figure 10-6 shows how the admissions from members of the medical staff might be forecast. At this point it is essential that the clinical manager and/or the individual physicians who will be accountable for the forecast admissions assist in the preparation of this forecast and agree to be accountable for the volume of admissions forecast.

To assist the clinical manager during the period covered by the forecast, a monthly report such as that shown in figure 10-7 might be appropriate. Comments from the clinical manager explaining the reason for the variances and what action is being taken to meet the forecast would be helpful in the ongoing process of managing according to the desired result for the budget year. To be of any assistance to the clinical manager in the reforecasting of patient volume for the remaining months, this report must be prepared, distributed, and analyzed on a timely basis. A report such as this prepared two months after the end of each quarter may help explain what happened but will be of little help in the process of managing for results or managing according to the budget objectives for the budget year.

Outpatient Data

Outpatient statistics are harder to interpret and forecast because of the varying nature of services. Certain outpatient services, such as the emergency department, are available to the community at the same level throughout the year even though their utilization may fluctuate significantly.

The following guidelines for collecting and forecasting outpatient statistics are helpful when estimating revenue, evaluating staffing requirements, and meeting capital requirements:

- Outpatient statistics for ancillary services can be obtained by analyzing ancillary department services by type of patient (inpatient, outpatient, and so forth) according to data in billing files or, in some cases, by procedure code assigned by the ancillary department and used for billing.
- Emergency department statistics should be segregated from other types of outpatient statistics.
- If clinics are a major part of the hospital's operations, the statistics for the larger clinics should be maintained separately.

Figure 10-3. Sample Format for Analyzing and Reporting Forecast Patient Days by Service

General Hospital
Patient Days by Service—1992 Operating Budget

Service Year	Beds Available	Jan.	Feb.	Mar.	April	May	June
Medicine							
1989	76	2,159	2,016	2,207	2,141	2,167	2,064
1990	76	2,231	2,081	2,313	2,185	2,314	2,198
1991[a]	76	2,261	2,047	2,295	2,179	2,240	2,132
1992 budget	76	2,382	2,117	2,382	2,382	2,382	2,117
Surgery							
1989	98	2,541	2,541	2,859	2,541	2,859	2,859
1990	101[b]	2,660	2,660	2,660	2,660	2,993	2,660
1991[a]	101	3,082	2,723	3,066	2,740	3,049	2,740
1992 budget	101	2,758	2,758	3,102	2,758	3,101	3,101
Intensive care unit							
1989	12	262	258	260	265	255	257
1990	12	264	206	235	235	205	235
1991[a]	12	272	238	237	243	269	240
1992 budget	12	246	236	241	251	261	251
Cardiac care unit							
1989	6	133	134	134	134	150	134
1990	12[b]	275	246	276	246	275	246
1991[a]	12	273	243	273	237	273	234
1992 budget	12	285	253	286	253	286	253
Pediatrics							
1989	15	286	287	287	287	287	287
1990	15	243	277	311	311	277	277
1991[a]	15	242	242	242	242	242	241
1992 budget	15	243	243	243	243	243	243
Obstetrics							
1989	22	500	444	445	445	445	500
1990	22	387	386	443	443	553	443
1991[a]	22	497	442	497	442	442	442
1992 budget	22	443	388	443	443	499	443

[a]Months January through July 1991 represent actual patient days. August through December are shown at current budget level.
[b]Three new surgery beds and six new beds in the intensive care unit were put into service 1/1/90.

- If outpatient revenue is a major part of the hospital's revenue, emergency department or clinic admissions (as discussed in a previous section of this chapter) should be noted separately in the statistics.

A sample format for analyzing and forecasting outpatient visits is shown in figure 10-8. The budget director should compile the historical information by using actual numbers of visits through the most recent month and forecast statistics for the remaining months of the current year. In figure 10-8, acute care represents the nonemergency-type care provided for such problems as colds and minor bruises and is available to the community at a relatively low charge. The emergency department statistics shown in figure 10-8 relate to true emergency visits. If the hospital classifies its emergency department visits by severity and charges accordingly, it is appropriate to record and forecast these visits by similar classification. Changes in trends by type of visit may have a significant effect on both revenue and staffing.

Figure 10-3. (Continued)

July	Aug.	Sept.	Oct.	Nov.	Dec.	Yearly Total Patient Days	Average Occupancy (%)
2,101	2,066	1,984	2,159	2,101	1,940	25,105	90.5
2,262	2,285	2,048	2,256	2,222	2,013	26,408	95.2
2,248	2,242	2,143	2,271	2,203	2,120	26,381	95.1
2,117	1,852	2,117	2,382	2,117	2,117	26,464	95.4
2,541	2,859	2,541	2,541	2,541	2,541	31,764	88.8
2,993	2,993	2,660	2,993	2,660	2,660	33,252	90.2
3,082	2,740	2,806	2,740	2,740	2,740	34,248	92.9
3,101	2,758	2,758	2,758	2,758	2,758	34,469	93.5
260	295	292	293	260	293	3,250	74.2
264	293	235	293	235	235	2,935	67.0
240	268	243	240	270	240	3,000	68.5
251	260	260	250	261	241	3,009	68.7
150	150	134	150	134	134	1,671	76.3
246	246	246	276	246	246	3,070	70.1
272	243	256	243	243	245	3,035	69.3
253	286	253	253	253	253	3,167	72.3
323	323	323	323	287	286	3,586	65.5
311	311	311	311	243	277	3,460	63.2
273	273	243	273	273	242	3,028	55.3
243	273	274	274	274	243	3,039	55.5
445	499	500	444	445	445	5,557	69.2
497	498	498	498	443	443	5,532	68.9
493	442	446	498	442	442	5,525	68.8
499	499	499	499	443	443	5,541	69.0

Figure 10-4. Sample Format for Analyzing and Reporting Forecast Facility Utilization

General Hospital
Analysis of Facility Utilization—1992 Operating Budget

Service[a]/Year	Type of Accommodations Available				Patient Days			
	1 Bed	2 Beds	Other	Total	1 Bed	2 Beds	Other	Total
Medicine								
1990	22	54	—	76	7,830	18,578	—	26,408
1991	22	54	—	76	7,880	18,501	—	26,381
1992	22	54	—	76	7,870	18,594	—	26,464
Surgery								
1990	17	80	4	101	5,840	26,682	730	33,252
1991	17	84	—	101	5,865	28,383	—	34,248
1992	17	84	—	101	5,865	28,604	—	34,469
(more)								

[a]Selected services for example only.

Figure 10-5. Sample Format for Analyzing Medical Staff Admissions

General Hospital
Physician Admission by Service—Actual 1990 Results

Service	Physician Admissions	Emergency Department	Metro Health Plan	Other Managed Care	Total
Medicine (including cardiac care)	3,546	119	140	48	3,853
Surgery (including intensive care)	3,934	137	179	52	4,302
Pediatrics	373	71	40	32	516
Obstetrics	985	17	135	65	1,202
Total	8,838	344	494	197	9,873

Figure 10-6. Sample Format for Forecasting Admissions by Physician

General Hospital
Forecast Admissions by Physician or Physician Group[a]

Surgery Admissions	1990	1991	Budget 1992	
			Range	Median
R. Evans	202	156	190−211	200
H. Brown[b]	60	44	—	—
F. Stein[c]	225	237	240−280	260
E. Moss	89	72	70−95	82
T. Alverez	57	67	55−70	62
A. Michael[c]	32	42	30−50	40
P. Phillips	72	64	60−70	65
L. Shapiro[c]	23	41	25−50	37
S. Rothman[d]	43	62	120−40	130
P. Fisher	115	132	115−135	125
Other surgeons (summarized for example)	2,015	2,935	2,568−3,201	3,001
Total	2,933	3,852	3,473−4,302	4,002

[a]Schedule excludes admission through emergency department or by HMO payers.
[b]Dr. H. Brown is turning over his practice to Dr. Stein and Dr. Phillips.
[c]Physicians practice together as Lakeshire Surgery Ltd.
[d]Dr. Rothman will perform a greater share of his total cases at General Hospital in 1992.

Figure 10-7. Sample Format for Monitoring Physician Admissions

General Hospital
Monthly Analysis of Hospital Admissions by Physician—January through March 1992

| Surgeon | Budget 1992 | | Actual Admissions[a] | | |
	Expected Range	Median	To Date	Annualized	Variance (Unfavorable)
R. Evans	190–200	200	32	167	(33)
H. Brown	—	—	—	—	—
F. Stein	240–280	260	80	280	20
E. Moss	70–95	82	18	78	(4)
T. Alverez	55–70	62	19	70	8
A. Michael	30–50	40	18	76	36
P. Phillips	60–70	65	20	72	7
L. Shapiro[b]	25–50	37	12	42	5
S. Rothman	120–140	130	32	128	(2)
P. Fisher	115–135	125	28	112	(13)
G. Samuels[c]	—	—	10	40	40
Others	2,568–3,201	3,001	713	2,689	(312)
Total	3,473–4,302	4,002	982	3,754	(248)

[a]Annualized admissions based on 1991 monthly admission trend.
[b]Dr. Shapiro was on vacation for the month of September.
[c]Dr. Samuels is a new member of Lakeshire Surgery Ltd.

Ancillary Department Statistics

Because ancillary services are an important part of total revenue, it is essential to have a sound projection of ancillary department statistics on which to base revenue estimates and develop resource requirements for generating that revenue. Because changes in ancillary revenue are a function of the type (mix) of services offered, the volume (intensity) of the services, and the price of the services, it is desirable to develop statistics that are based on changes in mix and intensity as reflected in the forecast admissions by program.

Methods of Estimating Utilization

Several different methods may be used to estimate ancillary utilization, depending on the information available. Projections can be based on any of the following:
- Current inpatient ancillary charges for each department per patient day or per admission adjusted for a utilization factor that is based on historical trends and known changes in services of the department (historical ancillary utilization can be measured in terms of dollars or the average number of services per patient day or per admission)
- Historical weighted average number of procedures in each ancillary department related to patient days or admissions (weighted procedure volume is determined on the basis of the relative work-load requirements for each procedure performed by the department and the volume of each procedure performed in prior periods)
- Historical trend for individual procedures in each ancillary department adjusted for anticipated changes in the volume and mix of patients resulting from the program forecast and analysis

Figure 10-8. Sample Format for Analyzing Outpatient Visits

General Hospital
Outpatient Visits by Service—1992 Operating Budget

| Service[a]/Year | Number of Visits by Month | | | | | | | | | | | | Total Visits |
	Jan.	Feb.	March	April	May	June	July	Aug.	Sept.	Oct.	Nov.	Dec.	
Emergency department													
1990	562	465	536	598	650	668	699	754	696	641	531	549	7,349
1991 (projected)	560	466	513	587	644	684	728	785	720	660	520	560	7,427
1992 (budget)	550	460	505	575	635	675	720	770	710	510	550	650	7,310
Acute care													
1990	111	92	101	112	122	125	132	136	131	114	99	104	1,379
1991 (projected)	148	98	161	152	155	156	135	150	140	130	130	120	1,675
1992 (budget)	180	125	195	185	190	190	165	180	170	160	155	145	2,040

[a]Selected patient services for example only. Ambulatory surgery would be a separate category. A separate analysis of each different type of ambulatory service would be useful for determining revenue and monitoring program trends identified in strategic goals and projections.

The most basic method of estimating utilization is to analyze and project statistics on the basis of monthly trends in numbers of procedures performed or trends of utilization per patient admission. This requires only that an analysis be prepared that shows the total number of procedures performed each month in each ancillary department. When this method is used, it is helpful to analyze all ancillary departments by month, as shown in figure 10-9, to relate the monthly utilization in each department to the other departments as well as to forecast admissions by month. Figure 10-9 shows only two ancillary services as examples. These two services, laboratory and diagnostic radiology, perform procedures that are relatively easy to identify from billing information. Statistics on the hours or minutes of operating room time, possibly by class of surgery, would be more difficult to obtain if methods for surfacing the statistics were not built in to the charge structure. In any case, the analysis should identify the statistic used. It is also necessary to choose the source for this type of statistic. Should it be records kept by the department, or should it be statistics based on billed charges? Commonly, the difference between these sets of data can be accounted for by lost charge slips, charge slips uncounted because of incorrect patient number, procedures performed for quality control, and performance of ancillary procedures still in development for which there is no charge. *Because ancillary service statistics are being used primarily to develop hospital revenue and also to measure productivity, it is appropriate to use the number of procedures billed because that statistic is usually more reliable.*

An alternative method of analyzing and forecasting the same data would be to show utilization per admission for each ancillary department. A sample format is shown in figure 10-10. As in the case of the monthly analysis, these statistics are projected on the basis of historical trends adjusted for changes in intensity and for the addition of specific new services. Intensity measures the growth in volume generated, not by increased admissions but by the greater number of services provided to each patient. When diagnostic program information is available, this analysis should be further broken down to reflect expected utilization for similar types of patients (as defined by program or similar clinical patient grouping). For example, the pharmacy department might expect to dispense more or different medications than in prior years because of a change in the program mix of patients. Relating expected pharmacy resource requirements to anticipated admission of specific types of patients would also help manage actual resource requirements during the budget year.

In either method, the historical portion of the analysis is performed by the budget director or by another staff member under his or her supervision. The projection for the budget period is developed by administrative staff and technical personnel in the appropriate departments.

It is suggested that the historical portion in several of the schedules described in this chapter be completed by the budget director because it is helpful to have the historical data consistently calculated from the same data base. A computer-based system can help provide this information. Several computer programs are available for mainframe, minicomputer, personal computer, or time-share applications. The historical data required for these analyses are typically available from the hospital's computerized billing files.

Relative Value Units

Basically, relative value units represent an indexing technique for relating work effort to output. Relative value units are used as a measure of output and are particularly helpful in determining work load, measuring productivity, and calculating procedure costs in service areas such as the laboratory or radiology. They are typically used to

Figure 10-9. Sample Format for Analyzing and Forecasting Ancillary Procedures by Service

General Hospital
Ancillary Procedures by Service—1992 Operating Budget

Service[a]/Statistic	Jan.	Feb.	March	April	May	June	July	Aug.	Sept.	Oct.	Nov.	Dec.	Total	Breakdown of Total Inpatient	Outpatient
Laboratory (tests billed)															
1990	22,479	24,063	20,752	25,761	25,559	23,257	23,947	22,912	24,897	24,782	25,387	24,034	297,830	207,792	80,038
1991 (projected)[b]	21,872	27,496	22,530	28,424	24,444	22,440	24,983	23,277	27,017	26,870	25,342	24,505	299,200	216,000	83,200
1992 (budget)	25,020	31,455	25,773	30,805	28,648	26,697	28,237	26,971	30,907	30,051	29,676	28,035	342,275	255,130	87,145
Diagnostic radiology (procedures billed)															
1990	1,509	1,422	1,586	1,536	1,715	1,753	1,800	1,731	1,671	1,470	1,511	1,613	19,317	11,775	7,542
1991 (projected)[b]	1,693	1,471	1,653	1,608	1,701	1,712	1,879	1,818	1,749	1,686	1,537	1,573	20,080	12,240	7,840
1992 (budget)	1,758	1,655	1,847	1,788	1,999	2,044	2,097	2,015	1,946	1,712	1,760	1,879	22,500	13,921	8,579

[a]Ancillary services shown here are for example only.
[b]The current year, 1991, includes actual procedures through July. August through December are projected at current budget levels.

Figure 10-10. Sample Format for Analyzing and Forecasting Inpatient Ancillary Procedures per Admission

General Hospital
Inpatient Ancillary Procedures per Admission

Services[a] (Statistic)	1989	1990	1991	1992
Operating room (half-hour increments)	0.935	0.960	1.009	1.171
Radiology (procedures)	1.092	1.123	1.237	1.430
EKG (procedures)	0.930	0.957	0.995	1.137
Nuclear medicine (procedures)	0.059	0.061	0.064	0.075

[a]Selected ancillary services for example only.

weight procedure volumes, as indicated in a previous section of this chapter, to more appropriately determine resource requirements. The compilation of relative value units for a particular department provides a basis for the following:

- Projecting the work load of the department and using that projection to estimate staffing requirements
- Measuring the changes in the department's weighted output (productivity) from period to period
- Developing the cost of various diagnostic or treatment procedures performed by the department

The use of relative values is helpful in establishing procedure charges based on the full cost of the individual procedure and in budgeting and controlling labor costs.

There are several resources for determining relative values for individual procedures:

- Values published by recognized entities such as the Canadian standards for radiology, the College of American Pathology standards for the laboratory, or the Hospital Association of New York standards for many hospital departments
- Engineering studies that measure the time required to perform each test within a department of the hospital

Relative values, regardless of how they were determined, are used to allocate applicable resources. The studied time requirements for each test and the expected volume of each test in a department are used to allocate the labor budgeted to provide all tests. There is an important distinction between allocation and standard buildup. In the allocation process, one begins with the budgeted labor. In the standard buildup process, one begins with the time requirement for each test, the productivity factors, and the expected volume for each test and determines what the budgeted labor should be. Both methods might result in "budget standards," but the results might be significantly different.

Relative values used together with a good department budget to develop budget standards have the advantage of providing realistic but challenging standards for all procedures at a reasonable level of effort. Because of the importance of determining a total cost for treating an individual patient, it is important that each and every procedure be costed.

Allocation rather than specific cost buildup is appropriate because the maintenance of actual cost as well as budgeted cost is at the department or cost-center level, not at the procedure level. In any one department, each person will perform various procedures but will not keep track of his or her time by procedure. Budget standards based on allocated costs will provide the basis for variance analysis at the department level (as was described in an earlier chapter).

Figure 10-11 demonstrates how relative value units are used in a system to establish procedure prices based on the full cost of individual procedures. The example uses only a few hematology tests; however, the methodology can be applied to all procedures performed by the department. The total allocated costs shown in the figure are adjusted to reflect the hospital's full financial requirements for replacement and growth. The calculation in figure 10-11 allocates each direct and indirect cost associated with the operation of the laboratory to the tests on the basis of specified statistics. All costs related to a particular test are added to arrive at the full cost of performing the test. The cost category in each column is either fixed or variable. This determination is necessary for the development of a department budget that flexes based on the actual volume and mix of the procedures performed. Actually, the calculation is performed by a computer program that uses budgeted cost and volume information and applicable procedure-level statistics for each category of costs. Each column in figure 10-11 is explained in the following paragraphs.

Column 1, **relative value unit,** represents the amount of direct technical labor time required to perform the test. The time requirements for each test are calculated by laboratory personnel on the basis of time studies and industry standards for the test. Rather than the time to build up a standard procedure cost, the time requirement for each test together with the volume of each test is used to allocate the total budgeted direct labor cost to each of the procedures.

Column 2, **projected volume,** represents an estimation of the number of tests to be performed within the coming year. Projections are calculated by each department on the basis of historical trend analysis and are adjusted to reflect upcoming program changes.

Column 3, **direct labor,** includes those labor costs in the department that are directly related to providing the individual service, procedure, or test. The direct labor costs are variable in that they are expected to vary in direct proportion to changes in volume of each procedure. In the laboratory, the direct labor category would include most of the labor cost for laboratory technicians and medical technologists. Direct

Figure 10-11. Calculation of Full Cost of Ancillary Procedures Based on Relative Value Units

General Hospital
Laboratory Tests—1992 Operating Budget

Test Code	Description[a]	[1] Relative Value Unit	[2] Projected Volume (# tests)	[3] Direct Labor	[4] Indirect Labor	[5] Overtime	[6] Direct Supply
51156	Cyto study blood	19.45	5	$ 5.77	$13.75	$1.21	$1.00
51157	Cyto study marrow	58.33	17	17.30	41.24	3.63	1.00
51168	Sucrose lypis	17.50	5	5.19	12.37	1.09	2.00
55011	Cell count	8.56	8	2.54	6.05	0.53	0.25
56011	Urinalysis	1.99	16,020	0.59	1.40	0.12	0.34
59011	Gastric analysis	3.88	16	1.15	2.75	0.24	0.25
61011	Feces standard	1.96	695	0.58	1.37	0.12	0.17
61013	Fat feces	2.33	70	0.69	1.65	0.15	0.29
63011	CBC—automated	2.90	26,280	0.86	2.05	0.18	—
63011	CBC—manual	5.43	3,030	1.61	3.85	0.34	1.09
63013	Model S	1.35	6,360	0.40	0.95	0.08	0.29
63017	Reticulocytes—automated	2.02	4,000	0.60	1.44	0.13	0.44
63022	Platelets ZBI	2.43	8,940	0.72	1.70	0.15	0.73
63023	Eosinophil	2.33	290	0.69	1.65	0.15	0.22
63025	Sedimentation rate	1.18	1,300	0.35	0.82	0.07	0.04
63027	Sickle cell	0.76	1,420	0.23	0.55	0.05	0.95

[a]Selected tests for example only.

labor cost per test is computed by multiplying direct labor time per test (the relative value for labor) by the average direct labor rate per relative value unit. The rate per unit is calculated by dividing the total budgeted direct labor dollars by the total relative value units. Total relative value units are the sum of the relative value for each procedure times the budgeted volume for each test. Because these costs are variable, it should be expected that for each additional cyto study blood performed by the laboratory, an additional $5.77 of direct labor would be required. The total dollar amount for direct labor varies according to the volume of each test.

Column 4, indirect labor, includes the department labor costs that do not vary directly with volume. Examples might be a department manager or a secretary. The costs do not vary directly with the volume of each test. The indirect labor costs in this example were allocated using the direct labor relative value unit, and they might also have been allocated to each test equally. Also, because the cost does not vary with the volume, the total indirect labor is expected to remain the same as the department volume varies. As a result of volume changes, the amount applicable to each test will vary. As the total department volume increases, the amount of indirect labor allocated to each procedure will decrease.

In **Column 5, overtime,** total hours and the aggregate cost are estimated by the department. Relative value units were the basis for overtime allocation to individual tests.

Column 6, direct supply, is a variable cost. The relative value for allocating the budgeted department direct supply cost should be based on actual recent purchases of supplies that relate to each procedure. The direct supply cost per test should be updated each year to reflect changes in individual supply prices and the supply amounts used for each test. Once again, because the recent supply costs are used to allocate the total department supply costs, a good test of reasonableness is simply a comparison of the relative value unit to the cost allocated to each individual procedure.

Figure 10-11. (Continued)

[7] Indirect Supply	[8] Allocated Cost	[9] Equipment Depreciation	[10] Outside Service Cost	[11] Total Test Cost	[12] Other Financial Considerations	[13] Total Cost (Cols. 11 and 12)	[14] Price (as of 1/1/92)	[15] Variance (Price − Cost)
$0.55	$18.75	$ —	$—	$ 41.03	$1.63	$ 42.66	$ 50.00	$ 7.34
0.55	56.25	—	—	119.97	4.26	124.23	150.00	25.77
0.55	16.87	—	—	38.07	1.40	39.47	40.00	.53
0.55	8.25	—	—	18.16	0.67	18.83	14.00	(4.83)
0.55	1.91	—	—	4.91	0.18	5.09	6.50	1.41
0.55	3.75	—	—	8.69	0.35	9.04	8.00	(1.04)
0.55	1.87	—	—	4.66	0.17	4.83	6.00	1.17
0.55	2.25	—	—	5.57	0.19	5.76	4.00	(1.76)
0.55	2.80	0.11	—	6.54	0.23	6.77	10.00	3.23
0.55	5.25	0.11	—	12.79	0.46	13.25	12.00	(1.25)
0.55	1.30	0.11	—	3.67	0.13	3.80	5.00	(1.20)
0.55	1.96	—	—	5.11	0.18	5.29	7.00	1.71
0.55	2.32	0.05	—	6.21	0.22	6.43	7.00	0.57
0.55	2.25	—	—	5.50	0.20	5.70	5.00	(0.70)
0.55	1.12	—	—	2.95	0.11	3.06	5.00	1.94
0.55	0.75	—	—	3.07	0.11	3.18	5.00	1.82

Column 7, **indirect supply,** is a fixed cost representing department supplies that do not vary directly with changes in procedure volume. In the example, indirect supply costs were allocated equally to each procedure. Office supplies are an example of an indirect supply cost.

Column 8, **allocated cost,** is usually regarded as fixed institutional support or overhead costs allocated to the department using the relevant statistics for each type of cost. Housekeeping might, for example, be allocated to the departments cleaned on the basis of floor space. Supporting schedules for this type of calculation should identify the institutional overhead expense categories and their bases of allocation. Department-allocated costs are assigned to each test equally when management feels that the allocated costs will not vary in direct proportion to changes in volume.

Column 9, **equipment depreciation,** which is fixed cost for specific procedures, is calculated on the basis of the following information submitted by the department:

- Which tests use the machine
- How much machine time each test takes
- How many tests are performed per year

Thus, the tests that use the equipment are responsible for and are assigned the related depreciation. Because the depreciation is fixed for a specific procedure or set of procedures, the amount allocated to the applicable procedure will vary according to the volume of that procedure.

Column 10, **outside service cost,** reflects any variable costs that are incurred outside of the laboratory and are needed to perform the procedure. Expenses are allocated to the individual test for which the outside service cost is incurred.

Column 11, **total test cost,** represents the total allocated cost for each test as determined by this methodology on the basis of the assumed volumes.

Column 12, **other financial considerations,** represents the hospital's fixed working capital and cash-flow requirements for the coming year. The costs are allocated to each department on the basis of the department's percentage of the institution's total direct expense. The amount of other financial requirements is proposed by the fiscal services department but must be reviewed and approved by the budget committee. For the purposes of the price and cost analysis, the departmental total for other financial considerations was allocated to each test on the basis of its percentage of total test costs, shown in column 11.

Column 13, **total cost,** represents the sum of total test costs (column 11) and other financial considerations (column 12).

The data in column 14, price, are submitted by the laboratory to the budget director. The prices used in this analysis include the 1992 increases.

Column 15, **variance,** is the difference between the price and total cost.

Statistical Applications to Information for Department Resource Management

When the institution puts the preceding year's statistics for patient days and ancillary procedures (as well as dollars) in the form of the program matrix shown in chapter 4, it can make statistical projections that include anticipated changes in admission by program. A statistical description showing days of stay in each type of patient unit (medical, surgical, intensive care, cardiac care, pediatrics, obstetrics/gynecology) and the procedures utilized in each ancillary unit can be developed for each admission in each program. A forecast of admissions by programs would therefore show the projected patient days in each one of the patient units and would project the utilization of each of the ancillary departments. The cost per procedure applied to each procedure budgeted for each program admission would enable management to predict cost by type of patient. Cost by type of patient is very useful for budgeting and managing resource utilization, for pricing contracts, and for managing actual resource utilization by contract.

The development of the statistics and the costs described in this chapter enable managers to develop and utilize the department information described in chapter 5. The process is not complicated. The calculations and the manipulation of department-level data can be supported by any one of a number of computer-based support systems available on the market. As described in chapter 5, this level of information is essential to the successful management of department-level resources.

Chapter 11

Revenue Budget

The revenue budget has become more important in recent years because management has less flexibility to maintain net income by adjusting rates. Contracts cover an increasing proportion of the total patients served. The contract rates are negotiated more frequently on the basis of a per case, per diem, or capitation method and less frequently on the basis of the charge structure. Once revenue is set, hospital management focuses on expense, which must be carefully managed to maintain net income. Because total revenue is less frequently the basis for charging patients, net revenue is determined by contract, and both total patient revenue and contractual allowances become less meaningful.

The revenue budget depends on the quality of the statistics gathered earlier in the budget cycle and the interpretation supplied by clinical, program, and department managers. Revenue is directly related to the volume and mix of patients served and the prices at which the services are contracted. Revenue projections are much more speculative than expense projections because a large proportion of expenses are related to personnel costs, which tend to be relatively constant. Variations of actual activity around projected activity may cause significant changes in revenue but not an equivalent change in the level of expense. Revenue is totally variable, but expenses are only partially variable. Whereas the relationship can offer opportunity in areas of growth, it can be a dilemma in areas of contraction. The necessity of management action to control costs in times of contraction also explains why no hospital cost is truly fixed. In the current environment, any cost, fixed or variable, can be reduced.

The rate structure and contract prices that support the revenue projection should be based on financial needs and expected volume and, therefore, usually will be reviewed several times throughout the budget process. As was discussed in chapter 8, the tentative or preliminary budget will reflect patient revenue based on budgeted statistics and current charge rates. Other revenue and operating expenses are reflected in the preliminary budget at the full budgeted amount. This format provides the basis for a reexamination of the rate increase and net income guidelines established at the beginning of the process, an analysis of the revenue requirements, and a determination of new rates for the budget year. As the revenue requirements and the general guidelines are reexamined, management should be provided with an update on conditions that might affect the budget decisions, such as changes in the state payment, status of current payer contract negotiations, and rates charged by other institutions in the community.

Management should also reexamine the requirement for an excess of revenue over expense so that the institution can meet the needs of ongoing operations. The importance of the operating margin or net income was discussed earlier in chapter 9. Throughout the budget process, from the development of the revenue budget to its final approval, the budget is constantly examined, and revenue and expenses are adjusted and balanced to ensure an adequate net income.

The actual development of the charge rates must be in accordance with the policies and guidelines established by management at the beginning of the budget cycle and updated before the development of the revenue budget. Rate development includes the following steps:

- Determination of the total financial requirements of the hospital according to the procedures described so far in this book
- Preparation of a cost-finding analysis on the basis of the statistics and expense projections for the budget year (this analysis identifies the total direct and indirect costs for each of the revenue-producing responsibility centers or departments; it also provides a basis for a pricing strategy that considers the utilization of each department by charge-paying patients)
- Establishment of a desired level of operating margin or net income for each responsibility center or department (at this point, management reviews historical trends, current environmental constraints, and regulatory constraints and decides the relative contribution of each responsibility center to the overall operating margin)
- Review of rates paid by Medicare, Medicaid, and other major contractors and calculation of the revenue expected from each major payer on the basis of projected contract rates and volume
- Review of expected changes in case mix and department volumes on the basis of the program analysis discussed in previous chapters
- Establishment of charge rates on the basis of direct costs, indirect costs as apportioned to the revenue centers through the cost-finding process, and desired contribution to the operating margin
- Review of the adequacy of the total revenue generated by the individual rates and the contract rates on the basis of total financial requirements

Because revenue results from a variety of activities, the revenue projection is developed for each activity individually. Generally, these activities include patient care (which encompasses daily nursing services, the basic daily charge), ancillary services, and other services that are indirectly related or somewhat unrelated to patient care (such as cafeteria, coffee shop, and gift shop). Revenue projections also include investment income (including changes in the market value of unrestricted investments), donations and grants, and income from tax levies.

All revenue is projected on a monthly basis. Monthly projections are useful for determining reasonableness (by comparing current experience and the actual experience of prior years) and for maintaining control during the budget year. Monthly projections are relatively easy to develop from statistics generated to this point in the budget process.

Patient Revenue

The largest single source of revenue is services provided to patients. Outpatient revenue is estimated on the basis of average revenue per type of visit using the statistics described earlier in chapter 10. An average is utilized because detailed outpatient statistics usually are not collected or analyzed in the same detail as inpatient statistics.

Outpatient statistics, however, should be collected in detail and maintained for program analysis along with inpatient statistics. In the current health care environment, outpatient services, such as ambulatory surgery, are replacing services that only a few years ago were provided on an inpatient basis. Now is the time for managers to keep and utilize better statistics on the outpatient services provided by the hospital.

The first step is to keep an accurate record of the total number of outpatient services by specific type of service. Typical types of outpatient services include emergency department visits, ambulatory surgery, and clinic visits. The second step is to utilize the charge system to track every specific charged service for an outpatient and, where the costs and other factors indicate, establish a different charge structure for outpatients.

In the past, the method of determining total patient revenue was to focus on the total charges and then calculate contractual allowances based on the payer mix. In the current environment, the use of contracts with specific payment provisions based on per case (diagnosis-related group [DRG]), per diem, or variable discounts makes it appropriate to calculate the total revenue, the discount, and the net revenue in a single calculation for each major payer. Each payer calculation should be separate, with the sum of the calculations providing the total inpatient revenue, total contractual allowances, and total net revenue for the hospital budget. This process also has the advantage of developing the information (described in chapter 7) required for effective program resource management.

An up-to-date budget process will reflect management's responsibility and accountability as described on a program and/or contract basis. The patient revenue in a hospital budget should be developed and analyzed by program, however defined, and by contract. A program analysis should be prepared to show the revenue in each program, broken down by contract. The format might be programs on the vertical axis of a matrix and contracts or payer types on the horizontal axis. The purpose of the analysis is to show the source of program revenue and relate the relative desirability of payer mix to each program.

The program analysis should be prepared in addition to the analysis of patient revenue by contract. The contract analysis shows the relative level of payment from each major payer. It relates directly to management's responsibility to negotiate effectively. When compared to prior years, the analysis reflects the payment trends of each major contractor.

Figure 11-1 illustrates how the total revenue could be summarized by payer. The payment rate for each payer is based on the terms of the contract. Medicare revenue, for example, is based on a per case calculation with a specific rate for each type of case as defined by DRG. The calculation is then adjusted for graduate medical education, patients using substantially more resources than the average (outliers), and other factors. Historical trends, program changes, contract limits, contract incentives, and so forth provide the basis for estimating the number of cases for each contract. The data used for estimating physician admissions by service (figure 10-5) are helpful in estimating the admissions and inpatient days by contract.

The calculation for the Medicaid contract can be based on a modified Medicare DRG, a per diem rate defined by type of service, or another calculation. The revenue, contractual allowance, and net revenue for Medicaid is calculated on the basis of estimated utilization and known contract terms. In the budget summary, the calculation could be summarized as shown in figure 11-1 to identify the contract revenue and the terms of the contract.

A significant contract with a health maintenance organization (HMO) (Metro Health Plan in the example) may be based on a capitation rate. The capitation rate is a set amount paid to the hospital for each person the hospital guarantees inpatient

Figure 11-1. Sample Format to Analyze Budget Revenue

General Hospital
Analysis of Budget Revenue by Payer

	Projected		Budget			Net Revenue
Payer	Discharges (Visits)	Patient Days	Total Revenue	Contractual Allowance	Net Revenue	as a Percentage of Total Revenue
Inpatient						
Medicare	2,689	21,511	$ 7,467,320	$1,650,104	$ 5,817,216	77.9%
Medicaid	2,075	14,110	4,267,040	1,706,816	2,560,224	60.8
Metro Health	683	4,781	1,866,830	300,913	1,565,917	83.9
Blue Cross	714	5,498	1,866,830	237,087	1,629,743	87.3
Commercial[a]	3,311	25,491	9,334,150	103,080	9,231,070	98.9
Other	566	4,298	1,866,830	—	1,866,830	100.0
	10,038	75,689	$26,669,000	$3,998,000	$22,671,000	85.0
Outpatient	32,509	—	3,576,000	207,000	3,369,000	94.2
Total	—	—	$30,245,000	$4,205,000	$26,040,000	86.1%

[a]Commercial includes managed care contracts.

services, regardless of how much each person uses the hospital resources during the contract period. In the Metro Health Plan calculation, the net revenue would be equal to the capitation rate times the number (and type) of enrollees covered. The total patient revenue would be the charges for the total of expected services required by patients covered by the HMO. Total patient revenue based on hospital charges might be helpful in analyzing resource usage, but total revenue would not affect contracted revenue for services to capitation patients.

The preceding examples point out the increasing importance of net revenue, the contract price, or the amount that the contractor is expected to pay. As the percentage of total hospital services covered by contracts (such as those based on a per case, per diem, or per capita calculation) increase, the relevance of the revenue recorded based on a full charge decreases. The relevance of the total revenue by department also decreases and may even become misleading. Instead of developing more hospital net income by increasing the number of procedures for each patient, the department may really be reducing the hospital net income by incurring additional expenses but not developing any additional revenue.

Two fundamental changes should occur when contracts such as those described represent a significant portion of the hospital's business. The first change is to report net revenue instead of total revenue as the top line of the published income statement. Contractual allowances or discounts should not be shown on the statement. For example, a major automobile company would not show revenue based on the sticker price of the automobiles sold and would not reflect fleet discounts, sales promotions, and other discounts as an offset to the sticker price revenue in its published financial statements. Showing total revenue and contractual allowances also heightens the awareness among some payers of how much more they are paying than other payers.

The second change is to stop reporting revenue by department. Senior management is responsible for successfully negotiating and managing the contracts. Department managers are responsible for managing hospital resources effectively on the basis of the volume and mix of services ordered by physicians. Senior managers, clinical managers, contract managers, or program managers are responsible for monitoring actual physician order patterns against the expected order patterns for contract patients.

If the budget manager were unable to manipulate procedure volumes as a means of estimating revenue, an alternative would be to use the historical correlation of specific ancillary utilization to key statistics such as surgery admissions, emergency department admissions, and obstetrics admissions. Having this type of detailed information facilitates a specific ancillary revenue projection that identifies volume changes by procedures and the effect of new procedures. Ancillary revenue variances during the budget year can then be easily identified and linked to changes in specific types of patients.

Once the detailed analyses have been completed, the budget committee must determine whether the result is reasonable. A schedule that pulls together the revenue calculations and shows the change in revenue due to rate change and volume is helpful. If the hospital were not utilizing program management, the format in figure 11-2 would be useful. If the hospital had the capability to analyze revenue by program, a further analysis in the format of figure 7-3 would be helpful in identifying the clinical services that create the demand for the resources of each patient care department.

Intensity

Intensity is the ancillary volume change, or the change in the average ancillary charge per patient day, that is due to a greater number of procedures per patient, not to a greater number of patients. As the average length of stay decreases, the intensity of ancillary services per patient day increases. The shorter length of stay has an impact on the profitability of a per diem contract. Intensity as measured on a per case basis could change as a result of a change in patient mix to a more acute level of care, the introduction of new technology, or changes in physician order patterns for the same patient types. Intensity could also be expected to increase as the less acute patients are more frequently treated on an outpatient basis. Because of the impact of intensity on the profitability of per case and per diem contracts, any increase in the average ancillary service volume per patient day or per admission should be determined and analyzed. Figure 11-2 provides the information needed to perform the per diem and per admission calculations. More detailed analyses of intensity can be developed around the patient resource information described in chapter 6. Hospital physicians should be directly involved in the analysis of intensity both to provide their knowledge of current practice and to increase their understanding of the impact of intensity on the profitability of current payer contracts. If the intensity factor cannot be explained by changes in program mix or new technology, the ancillary department-level projections should be reexamined.

Other Operating Income

Other operating income is part of total operating revenue. Related expenses, where expenses exist, are included in the total operating expenses of the hospital. Most revenue projections for these items can be broken down to volume and price.

Cafeteria and coffee shop revenue is a function of the prices charged and the number of employees and guests served. The budgeted revenue is based on historical volume and current average price per serving and adjusted for projected changes in the number of employees (from the personnel budget) and prices.

Gift shop revenue is estimated by the gift shop manager, who also knows of changes in the mix of merchandise that may change total revenue.

Revenue from telephone services, medical record reprints, and miscellaneous services is based on historical experience and adjusted for anticipated price changes.

Nonoperating Revenue and Expenses

Nonoperating revenue and expenses are shown separately on the income statement. They contribute to the net income (total resources) of the hospital. Unrestricted gifts and donations are probably the largest item and are estimated by the development officer and the chief executive officer. Investment income is projected on the basis of management's estimate of funds available for investment and future interest rates. After the cash budget is completed, this estimate may be revised.

Allowances for Third-Party Payers

A deduction from total patient revenue is necessary because most contract third-party payers pay less than charges for services to covered patients. Because services rendered

Figure 11-2. Schedule for Analyzing and Forecasting Inpatient Revenue According to Service

General Hospital
Inpatient Revenue Analysis—1992 Budget

Service	Statistic	Projected Volume 1991	Budget Volume 1992	Current Average Rate/Statistic
Medicine	Patient days	26,381	26,464	$116.00
Surgery	Patient days	34,248	34,469	116.00
Intensive care unit	Patient days	3,000	3,009	214.00
Cardiac care unit	Patient days	3,035	3,167	214.00
Pediatrics	Patient days	3,028	3,039	116.00
Obstetrics	Patient days	5,525	5,541	116.00
Nursery	Patient days	2,570[a]	2,502[a]	68.00
Average/total basic daily hospital charges		75,217[a]	75,689[a]	$126.18
Operating room	Patients	5,784	5,766	$232.46
Recovery room	Patients	5,304	5,346	45.61
Delivery room	Patients	1,683	1,679	138.60
Central supply	Requisitions[b]	156,591	157,391	6.22
Intravenous therapy	Charges	57,547	59,750	10.62
Emergency department	Visits	8,835	8,886	30.97
Anesthesiology	Patients	6,752	6,645	21.92
Day surgery	Patients	43	85	47.00
Laboratory	Tests	142,982	144,842	12.61
Blood bank	Charges	9,041	8,757	29.20
Electrocardiogram	Examinations	5,550	5,577	39.82
Cardiac catheterization lab	Examinations	413	455	634.78
Radiology	Examinations	21,944	20,972	31.58
Ultrasound	Examinations	213	214	112.50
Electroencephalogram	Examinations	411	413	97.32
Respiratory therapy	Treatments	41,216	41,167	10.53
Physical therapy	Treatments	16,788	16,929	12.39
Pharmacy	Doses	710,909	717,742	1.65
Nuclear medicine	Examinations	752	776	146.32
CT scan	Examinations	1,099	1,133	189.19
Average/total ancillary charges				
Average/total hospital charges				

[a]Reported patient days normally refer to adult and pediatric patients. Nursery days are shown but not included in average basic daily charge calculation.
[b]Includes surgical supplies for operating room.

to all patients are recorded in total patient service revenue at the full charge rates, an allowance is needed to reduce the gross revenue to the net amount that can be expected from the Medicare, Medicaid, and other programs that receive a discount.

Because of the many different contract terms and calculations and the relevance of the mix of payers in each revenue department, the best method for budgeting allowances is to perform an individual revenue calculation by using budget information for each of the payer programs. Previous sections in this chapter contain suggestions for showing the summary results of these calculations. It is important that the budget committee understand the terms of major contracts and that it is able to determine the reasonableness of the contractual allowance for each contract group.

The statistics generated in chapter 10 are very important for these calculations. The impact of any variance from the most recent actual experience should be carefully analyzed and explained.

Figure 11-2. (Continued)

Proposed Average Rate/Statistic	Percent of Change Due to Rate	Projected Revenue at Current Rates	Budget Revenue at Current Rates	Percent of Change Due to Volume	Budget Revenue Proposed Rates
$123.00	6	$ 3,060,196	$ 3,069,824	0.3	$ 3,255,072
123.00	6	3,972,768	3,998,404	0.7	4,239,687
226.00	6	642,000	643,926	0.3	680,034
226.00	6	649,490	677,738	4.2	715,742
123.00	6	351,248	352,524	0.4	373,797
123.00	6	640,900	642,756	0.3	681,543
70.00	3	174,760	170,136	(2.7)	175,140
$133.72	6.0	$ 9,491,362	$ 9,555,308	0.6	$10,121,015
$265.00	14	$ 1,344,548	$ 1,340,364	(0.3)	$ 1,527,990
52.00	14	241,915	243,831	0.8	277,992
158.00	14	233,263	232,709	(0.2)	265,282
6.90	11	973,996	978,972	0.5	1,085,997
12.00	13	611,149	634,545	3.8	717,000
35.00	13	273,619	275,199	0.6	311,010
25.00	14	148,003	145,658	(2.6)	166,125
47.00	—	2,021	4,000	99.7	3,995
14.25	13	1,803,003	1,826,458	1.3	2,063,998
33.00	13	263,997	255,704	(3.2)	288,981
45.00	13	221,001	222,076	0.5	250,965
730.00	15	262,164	288,825	10.2	332,150
36.00	14	692,991	662,296	(4.6)	754,992
126.00	12	23,962	24,075	0.3	26,964
109.00	12	39,998	40,193	0.5	45,017
12.00	14	434,004	433,489	(0.1)	494,004
14.00	13	208,003	209,750	0.8	237,006
1.86	13	1,172,999	1,184,274	1.0	1,335,000
161.00	10	110,062	113,575	3.2	124,936
210.00	11	207,919	214,352	3.1	237,930
	13.1	$ 9,268,617	$ 9,330,345	0.7	$10,547,334
	9.5	$18,759,979	$18,885,653	0.7	$20,668,349

Free Care and Uncollectible Accounts

The free care and uncollectible accounts revenue deduction category includes free care (defined as services to patients unable to pay), charity care provided in accordance with specific hospital services or agreements with specific donors, uncollectible accounts (defined as services to those who are able but unwilling to pay), and employee discounts. The total deduction must be a net amount. This means that the hospital must offset free care with donations that are restricted by the donor for the care of patients who are unable to pay. The provision for the cost of uncollectible accounts is an estimated amount, usually based on historical experience, that must be offset by amounts collected on accounts previously written off.

The amounts of these revenue deductions in the budget are subject to management's admitting and collection policies and are affected by changes in the economy that influence patients' ability to meet their financial obligations. The amounts should be budgeted on the basis of historical experience and adjusted for changes in policy, changes in payment provisions by major payers (an increase in the deductible and co-insurance provisions of a major payer could affect the expected uncollectible amount), and management's best guess as to changes in the economy that may affect patients' ability to pay. The basis for the calculation should be a comparison of actual experience for the past several years, shown as a dollar amount for each year and as a percentage of the applicable total patient service revenue and the net patient service revenue.

There sometimes may be a tendency not to record services that are provided without charge (free care) or at a discount. The correct procedure is to show the full charge in patient service revenue for every service performed and then show the full amount of free service or discount as a deduction. This procedure is correct for a number of reasons. All services require the use of hospital resources and are included in expense. The revenue for each department should relate directly to the amount of service provided. The statistics utilized to flex the expense budget for each department are based on charges. Not recording services results in an inaccurate, low-flexed budget with unfavorable variances and pressure on the department manager to reduce expenses to the flexed budget. Service cost cannot be related to charges if charges are not recorded. Finally, the hospital should get full credit in the community for free services provided to persons in the community. Free care cannot be documented if free services are not recorded.

In the analysis accompanying the budget presentation and in the calculation itself, uncollectible accounts are frequently shown as a percentage of total patient service revenue. As the percentage of patients covered by contracts increases, the comparison of uncollectible accounts to total patient service revenue misstates the impact of the uncollectible accounts. The budget calculation and the presentation should relate the amount uncollectible to the amount that should be collected from individual patients. When the hospital is collecting the contracted amounts from the third-party payers but only 50 percent of the amounts due from patients, that is the way it should be explained in the presentation.

Chapter 12

Personal Budget

Once the statistics have been gathered and analyzed and the revenue budget developed, the next step is to attach dollar amounts to the work-load requirements and prepare a budget of personnel costs and fringe benefits. Because salaries, wages, and fringe benefits represent more than 60 percent of the average hospital's total expense budget, it is important that personnel costs be carefully budgeted and controlled. Actually, the task of budgeting and controlling personnel costs is made easier by the fact that employees are easy to identify physically: each has a distinct name and number. The actual salary costs and statistics are readily available from routine payroll reports. In addition, employees tend to monitor their payroll checks carefully, and so the actual amounts shown in payroll records are generally accurate. The most important factor in controlling personnel costs, therefore, is not the amount of payroll being expended on current employees, but rather the establishment of a plan that shows which positions should be filled, when they should be filled, what the appropriate salary level for each position is, and what the expectations are for each position before it is filled.

Position Control System

Because managers at the department level are the individuals most effective in budgeting and controlling personnel costs, they should be provided with the tools to carry out that function. One such tool is a set of reasonable personnel policies for staffing, employment, termination, work-shift assignments, and determination of adequate salaries and wages. They should have the ability to set expectations, measure accomplishments, and reward results.

A second tool, which pertains to the control function, is the position control system. The documentation for this system is much like an expanded organizational chart in that it reflects every approved position, whether filled or vacant, in each responsibility center of the hospital. The position control system provides for a reasonable delegation of authority to line managers and offers a framework for evaluating the exercise of delegated authority. It is also an excellent basis for establishing the personnel budget.

When first establishing a position control system, it is necessary to identify each type of job that needs to be done within each responsibility center. The next step is to determine the skill levels within each general job description and the number of personnel required at each skill level to support the responsibility center's planned level of activity. As the job descriptions and the personnel requirements begin to take shape, the next step is to determine wage and salary ranges by using studies of the marketplace or existing wage and salary policy guidelines. The last step is matching employees with the positions described and recording individuals' names, wages or salaries, and other specific information.

Once the position control system is complete, hospital management has a complete outline of positions necessary in each responsibility center as well as authorized salary and hourly rate ranges. To be effective, however, the system must be kept up-to-date as hospital management approves positions to be added and eliminates others.

An example of a position control document form for an individual responsibility center is shown in figure 12-1. The number of personnel is expressed in terms of full-time equivalents, or the equivalent of a full-time position as defined by personnel policies. A fractional full-time equivalent indicates a part-time position.

The sample form in figure 12-1 has spaces for a labor grade classification code and description. A labor grade classification system assigns a code to each position in the personnel budget to assist management in establishing and controlling the personnel budget. Depending on the needs of management, the code may be used to designate various levels of information concerning the description and skill level of each position. Usually, this code designates wage and salary ranges as well as skill requirements. If it does not, a separate column can be used for approved wage and skill salary ranges.

The American Hospital Association's *Chart of Accounts for Hospitals* (Chicago: American Hospital Publishing, 1976) describes a system whereby the two digits to the right of the decimal in an account number are used to identify the type of expense by natural expense classification. Using this system, .01 represents employees with management and supervisory responsibilities; .02, technicians and specialists; .03, registered nurses; .04, licensed practical nurses; and so on. This system may be expanded to include more specific employee classifications. The classifications on the

Figure 12-1. Example of a Position Control Document for a Department

General Hospital
Approved Department Manpower

Date: _____   Page No.: _____
Department No.: _____   Department Name: _____

Labor Grade Classification (Job Code)[a]	Classification Description	Approved Full-Time Equivalents	Approved Wage/Salary Range[a]		Flexibility (%)	
			Annual	Hourly	Fixed	Variable

Wage-earning (hourly) full-time equivalents: _____
Administrative (salaried) full-time equivalents: _____
Total full-time equivalents: _____

[a]These columns must reflect the approved labor grade classification structure.

sample forms in this chapter use an expanded version of the American Hospital Association's classification system, which has been modified by adding slightly more detail for the nursing classifications.

At a certain level of detail, which depends largely on the institution's wage and salary policies, these codes can be used to represent salary ranges. For example, a specific code can represent a registered nurse category that has a specific salary range.

The benefits of this type of system include improved control over personnel budgets by management, which approves the labor grade classification rather than the salary for each person on the payroll. The initial effort required to determine the labor grade for each position and the ongoing review of each employee's qualifications as they relate to the labor grade classification's requirements are well worth the effort.

The form in figure 12-1 also contains a space for indicating the fixed or variable characteristic of each labor category. Those positions that depend directly on the level of department activity are described as variable. Those that are expected to remain constant are described as fixed. It is possible for a labor category to have both fixed and variable characteristics. For example, a nurse supervisor may have direct patient care and administrative responsibilities for the unit. The patient care position would be a part of the total unit's direct care requirements and would flex depending on patient days (and acuity). The administrative time would be expected to remain constant and would not be affected by the changes in patient days (or acuity).

Preparation of Personnel Budget

The development of the personnel budget depends on determining the number of workers at various skill levels who will be required to carry out the operating plan and the salary or wages they must be paid. The persons responsible for preparing the personnel budget are the line managers responsible for implementing the operating plan. They should have available to them the hospital's personnel policies, the position control documents for their departments or responsibility centers, information on current staffing, and appropriate budget work sheets. Personnel policies cover the methodology for determining appropriate wage and salary levels as well as policies on vacations, holidays, and other fringe benefits. The position control document shows positions currently approved for each responsibility center. Basically, the positions listed equal the preceding year's personnel budget plus or minus changes approved by management during the year. Figure 12-2 is an example of such a document, with additional space provided to summarize and explain changes for the upcoming budget.

When reviewing the level of staffing for assessing its reasonableness, budgeting fringe benefit expenses, or budgeting expenses for outside help, the fact that a hospital is a 24-hours-per-day, seven-days-per-week operation must be considered. For example, if the appropriate nurse staffing level for a particular unit were, on the average, three registered nurses for a given shift, the actual staffing required would be 4.2 registered nurses because of weekend staffing needs. Therefore, a factor of 1.4 is used to bring the five-days-per-week staffing level to seven days. In addition, consideration must be given to coverage for vacation days, holidays, and sick days. If proposed staffing does not adequately cover these periods, the cost of overtime or outside or temporary help should be included in the expense budget.

Positions shown in the position control document should also be reconciled with the current positions shown on payroll records to ensure that the control system is up-to-date and that current employees are properly classified. The updated position control system should also be reconciled to include positions requested for the budget period. To identify the actual staffing on a budget work sheet, it is helpful to have

Figure 12-2. Example of a Position Control Document for an Intensive Care Unit

General Hospital
Approved Department Manpower

Department: _____   No.: _____
Date Prepared: _____   Date Approved: _____
Approved: _____, Administrator
Approved: _____ Personnel Department

Code	Position Title	1990 FTE Budget	1991 FTE Budget	1991 FTE Budget	Difference
01	Registered nurse	15.00	16.00		
02	Nurse assistant	1.00	1.00		
03	Licensed practical nurse	2.00	3.00[a]		
04	Ward clerk	3.00	3.00		
06	Head nurse	3.00	3.00		
Total		24.00	26.00		

Comments: _____
_____
_____
_____
_____

[a]Full-time equivalent (FTE) approved during the year (2/11/91).

the appropriate line manager show the full-time equivalent positions for each shift within each labor grade classification. The line manager may be asked to complete a work sheet like the one shown in figure 12-3, as well as summary information on the position control document (figure 12-1). The historical and current staffing information needed to complete this form is supplied by the budget director to the line manager, who completes the form for the projected requirements.

If shift assignments are required for nursing or any other department, each shift should be shown separately on the work sheet, as in figure 12-3, and the personnel list for each shift should indicate job classifications separately. The individual classifications are important when the positions are translated to payroll costs because in most instances shift differentials or other incentives vary by classification.

Any increase or decrease from the current actual full-time equivalents to the full-time equivalent level requested for the budget period should be explained on the work sheet, on the summary form, or in an attachment. The approved positions for the budget period are the basis for updating position control documents and calculating the payroll costs to be reflected in the expense budget.

Most institutions rely on historical experience to determine required positions. When the information on the experiences of other hospitals is available from special services or hospital associations, most managers use it to make overall comparisons and determine reasonableness. When the institution has management-engineered standards, those standards can be used by line managers to determine staffing requirements and by the budget committee to review the requested positions.

Once the positions have been approved, the budgeted payroll expense can be calculated on the basis of actual salaries and wages for filled positions and the beginning-level salaries and wages for vacant positions. A schedule showing approved, current, and vacant positions and current annual salaries and wages for each responsibility unit should be prepared by the line manager. There should also be spaces to insert budgeted payroll expenditures by month.

As an alternative, the budget director can use the institution's classification system in the position control documents to project the hours required for each labor grade classification. Using this methodology, the differentials for such variables as overtime can be factored into the estimated requirements for full-time equivalents, and more detailed schedules need not be prepared. As described earlier in this chapter, line managers can reconcile the actual positions filled with the projected requirements by labor grade classification, using a format similar to that shown in figure 12-3.

When there is agreement on salary and wage increases, the budgeted total for each person should be distributed by month. Budgeted salaries or wages for vacant positions should begin in the month the line manager realistically believes the positions

Figure 12-3. Work Sheet for Documenting Past, Current, and Projected Personnel Needs for an Intensive Care Unit

General Hospital
Personnel Budget 1992

Approved: _____   Department: NURSING—INTENSIVE CARE UNIT 121
      (Administrator)
Approved: _____   Date: _____
      (Personnel)

Labor Grade Classification	1990 Budgeted FTE	1991 Budgeted FTE	1991 FTE Actual (as of 7/31/91)	Projected 1992 FTE
Shift 7:00 a.m.–3:00 p.m.:				
01 — Registered nurse	7.00	8.00	7.50	
02 — Nurse assistant	0.00	0.00	0.00	
03 — Licensed practical nurse	1.00	1.00	1.50	
04 — Ward clerk	1.00	1.00	1.00	
06 — Head nurse	1.00	1.00	1.00	
Total 7:00 a.m.–3:00 p.m.	10.00	11.00	11.00	
Shift 3:00 p.m.–11:00 p.m.:				
01 — Registered nurse	5.00	5.00	4.20	
02 — Nurse assistant	0.00	0.00	0.00	
03 — Licensed practical nurse	1.00	1.00	1.50	
04 — Ward clerk	1.00	1.00	1.00	
06 — Head nurse	1.00	1.00	1.00	
Total 3:00 p.m.–11:00 p.m.	8.00	8.00	7.70	
Shift 11:00 p.m.–7:00 a.m.:				
01 — Registered nurse	3.00	3.00	3.00	
02 — Nurse assistant	1.00	1.00	1.00	
03 — Licensed practical nurse	0.00	1.00	0.50	
04 — Ward clerk	1.00	1.00	1.00	
06 — Head nurse	1.00	1.00	1.00	
Total 11:00 p.m.–7:00 a.m.	6.00	7.00	6.50	
Total intensive care unit:				
01 — Registered nurse	15.00	16.00	14.70	
02 — Nurse assistant	1.00	1.00	1.50	
03 — Licensed practical nurse	2.00	3.00[a]	3.00	
04 — Ward clerk	3.00	3.00	3.00	
06 — Head nurse	3.00	3.00	3.00	
Total all shifts	24.00	26.00	25.20	

[a]Approved 1.00 FTE—2/11/91.

will be filled. Known terminations or retirements should also be reflected in the monthly amounts. Finally, the salaries and wages should reflect step and merit increases in the month they occur. For example, if the hospital's policy were to give a step increase to its employees at the beginning of the year and a merit increase to each individual employee on his or her anniversary date, these increases should be estimated and reflected in the appropriate month. A shift differential may be reflected in an individual employee's wages if the employee is permanently assigned to a shift, or it may be listed as a separate line item that is also spread by month if employees rotate through shifts.

The schedule format may follow the example shown in figure 12-4. In this example, it was assumed that the hospital management decided to budget a 4 percent step

Figure 12-4. Sample Format for Monthly Personnel Budget According to Job Classification

General Hospital
Personnel Budget by Job Classification—1992 Budget

Job Code	Authorized Positions	Current Rate per Hour[a]	Proposed Rate (effective 1/1/92)	Jan.	Feb.	March	April
01	B. Smith	$6.91	$7.19	$ 1,270	$ 1,147	$ 1,270	$ 1,229
	J. Aubin	6.09	6.33	1,118	1,009	1,118	1,082
	V. Jones	6.09	6.33	1,118	1,009	1,118	1,082
	R. James	6.58	6.84	1,208	1,091	1,208	1,169
	J. Short	6.75	7.02	1,240	1,120	1,240	1,200
	D. Clark	6.09	6.33	1,118	1,009	1,118	1,082
	G. Craig	6.41	6.67	1,132	1,025	1,132	1,140[b]
	S. Day	7.37	7.66	1,302	1,176	1,302	1,260
	T. Hall	7.04	7.32	1,243	1,123	1,243	1,205
	N. Lee	6.58	6.84	1,162	1,050	1,162	1,125
	D. Miller	6.75	7.02	1,192	1,080	1,192	1,154
	G. Bass	6.95	7.23	1,228	1,109	1,228	1,188
	P. Price	6.41	6.67	1,132	1,025	1,132	1,096
	H. Winter	6.58	6.84	1,162	1,052	1,162	1,159[b]
	Vacant	6.09	6.33	1,075	974	1,075	1,042
	Vacant	6.09	6.33	1,075	974	1,075	1,042
				$18,775	$16,973	$18,775	$18,255
02	P. Grady	3.95	4.11	$ 698	$ 630	$ 698	$ 675
03	P. Graf	4.63	4.82	$ 818	$ 736	$ 818	$ 792
	B. Hansen	4.91	5.11	867	784	867	840
	A. Anderson	4.80	4.99	848	764	848	821
				$ 2,533	$ 2,284	$ 2,533	$ 2,453
04	M. Hill	4.05	4.21	$ 715	$ 647	$ 715	$ 728[b]
	A. Jackson	3.88	4.04	685	619	685	667
	K. James	3.98	4.14	703	637	703	707[b]
				$ 2,103	$ 1,903	$ 2,103	$ 2,102
06	M. Taylor	7.23	7.52	$ 1,277	$ 1,190[b]	$ 1,277	$ 1,236
	B. Enton	7.36	7.65	1,300	1,177	1,300	1,258
	N. Hope	7.64	7.95	1,349	1,224	1,349	1,306
				$ 3,926	$ 3,591	$ 3,926	$ 3,800
	Totals			$28,035	$25,381	$28,035	$27,285

[a]Shift differential is 8 percent for evenings and 10 percent for nights. Holiday bonus is 10 percent for all shifts.
[b]Projected merit increase on anniversary date.

increase at the beginning of the year and an average merit increase of 4 percent to reward deserving employees on their individual anniversary dates. It also assumes that the wage rates include shift differentials. However, if nurses rotated through all three shifts, a separate budget amount should be calculated for the shift differentials and shown separately on the schedule. This institution also pays a bonus for working on Christmas Day and New Year's Day, and this bonus must be reflected in the budgets for January and December. The bonus is not shown on this schedule. Budgeted amounts for overtime or temporary help are included in a separate account and are not shown on these work sheets.

Another approach might be used to develop the personnel budget when the hospital's payroll data are computerized and can be tied to a computerized budget system.

Figure 12-4. (Continued)

Responsibility Unit: 121   Description: Intensive Care Unit

Prepared by: _____   Date: _____

May	June	July	Aug.	Sept.	Oct.	Nov.	Dec.	Total
$ 1,270	$ 1,229	$ 1,270	$ 1,321[b]	$ 1,278	$ 1,321	$ 1,278	$ 1,321	$ 15,204
1,118	1,082	1,174[b]	1,174	1,136	1,174	1,136	1,174	13,495
1,118	1,136[b]	1,174	1,174	1,136	1,174	1,136	1,174	13,549
1,208	1,169	1,208	1,256[b]	1,216	1,256	1,216	1,256	14,461
1,240	1,200	1,240	1,240	1,248[b]	1,290	1,248	1,290	14,796
1,118	1,136[b]	1,174	1,174	1,136	1,174	1,136	1,174	13,549
1,132	1,096	1,132	1,132	1,096	1,132	1,096	1,132	13,377
1,302	1,260	1,341[b]	1,302	1,260	1,302	1,260	1,302	15,369
1,243	1,240	1,243	1,243	1,205	1,243	1,205	1,243	14,679
1,197[b]	1,125	1,162	1,162	1,125	1,163	1,125	1,163	13,721
1,192	1,212[b]	1,192	1,192	1,154	1,192	1,154	1,192	14,098
1,228	1,188	1,228	1,277	1,188	1,228	1,188	1,227	14,505
1,132	1,096	1,132	1,132	1,129[b]	1,132	1,096	1,132	13,366
1,162	1,125	1,162	1,162	1,125	1,162	1,125	1,162	13,720
1,075	1,042	1,075	1,075	1,042	1,075	1,042	1,075	12,667
1,075	1,042	1,075	1,075	1,042	1,075	1,042	1,075	12,667
$18,810	$18,378	$18,982	$19,091	$18,516	$19,093	$18,483	$19,092	$223,223
$ 698	$ 675	$ 725[b]	$ 698	$ 675	$ 698	$ 675	$ 698	$ 8,243
$ 851[b]	$ 792	$ 818	$ 818	$ 792	$ 818	$ 792	$ 818	$ 9,663
867	840	867	911[b]	840	867	840	867	10,257
848	854[b]	848	848	821	848	821	848	10,017
$ 2,566	$ 2,486	$ 2,533	$ 2,577	$ 2,453	$ 2,533	$ 2,453	$ 2,533	$ 29,937
$ 715	$ 693	$ 715	$ 715	$ 693	$ 715	$ 693	$ 715	$ 8,459
685	663	712[b]	685	663	685	663	685	8,097
703	680	703	703	680	703	680	703	8,305
$ 2,103	$ 2,036	$ 2,130	$ 2,103	$ 2,036	$ 2,103	$ 2,036	$ 2,103	$ 24,861
$ 1,277	$ 1,236	$ 1,277	$ 1,277	$ 1,236	$ 1,277	$ 1,236	$ 1,277	$ 15,073
1,300	1,258	1,300	1,300	1,308[a]	1,300	1,258	1,300	15,359
1,349	1,345[b]	1,349	1,349	1,306	1,349	1,306	1,349	15,930
$ 3,926	$ 3,839	$ 3,926	$ 3,926	$ 3,850	$ 3,926	$ 3,800	$ 3,926	$ 46,362
$28,103	$27,414	$28,296	$28,395	$27,530	$28,353	$27,447	$28,352	$332,626

In this case, line managers can be given detailed work sheets showing filled and vacant positions, names, salaries, dates of hiring, and dates of next merit review. Each line manager is asked to review the information, reconcile it with that provided by position control documents, and return the work sheets to the budget director. The budget director then reviews all the differences identified and has the work sheets rerun with corrected information. Once the budget is final, line managers complete the forms to include authorized salary and wage increases, new positions, and upgraded positions. Each line manager also spreads the updated salary and wage information by position to the individual months before returning the corrected and updated work sheet to the budget director.

Staffing Variations

The examples in this chapter show the base staffing required for an expected level of activity. Because management must anticipate significant variations in utilization during the budget year, variable or step staffing is more appropriate. Variable staffing flexes the monthly staffing levels to forecasted units of service; for example, nurse staffing in each unit is tied to patient days (or patient days weighted by an acuity factor), and the laboratory technician staffing is tied to forecasted, weighted test statistics. During the budget year, the budget's staff-to-activity relationships will be used to flex the staffing budget to actual volumes. The flex-budget calculations require that each labor category be designated regarding its capacity to vary in direct proportion to changes in department activity. Some categories will have both a fixed component and a variable component because of the administrative or supervisory tasks performed, which do not vary directly with changes in patient care services.

In addition to the categories of fixed or variable cost, personnel requirements are analyzed in terms of step staffing. For example, the opening of a nursing unit would require a step-staffing approach. Opening and maintaining a unit at even the lowest level of utilization requires a core group of staff. Additional staff in the unit may be variable as the utilization increases, and so the budget staff requirements would increase over and above the core group. This step-staffing concept is an example of what is referred to as a relevant range in flexible budgeting. Any projection of the requirements is fixed or variable up to a point of increased or decreased utilization, at which the requirements should be reanalyzed and the fixed and variable components redefined. The change in patient days at some point requires the opening or closing of nursing units and the redefinition of nursing personnel requirements. If projected utilization covered several ranges of activity within a responsibility unit, the staffing should be budgeted and managed to reflect the changes in personnel requirements.

Whatever system is used to prepare the work sheets, the estimates of additional staff needed because of vacations, holidays, and overtime are shown separately on these or separate work sheets. The amounts budgeted for these expenses are not spread in the same ratio as salaries but follow previous experience for vacations taken, actual holidays, and current personnel policies.

Vacancy Allowance

After the personnel requirements have been estimated and the personnel costs calculated, an estimate is made of the costs that may not be incurred in the event of unforeseen turnover and vacant positions. In other words, the budget director, with the help of the line manager, estimates, as an offset to total salary and wage expenses, an amount that will probably not be paid because of normal turnover. Normal turnover reduces personnel expense requirements because a person leaving the department often leaves a position that remains vacant while a new employee is being sought and because the new employee is often hired at a salary level lower than that of the experienced person who left the position. The amount of the vacancy (or turnover) allowance is an educated guess based on past experience. It should be reviewed by the personnel department for reasonableness.

Fringe Benefits

Fringe benefits are closely related to personnel costs, employee statistics, and personnel policies. They are also difficult to budget accurately. Estimates of fringe benefits can be developed on the basis of past experience and adjusted for changes in regulations under the Federal Insurance Contributions Act (FICA), changes in pension and health care plans, and changes in other personnel policies. The hospital's insurance representative may also be able to provide assistance with some of the calculations. The usual list of fringe benefits would include:

- Employer's portion of Social Security taxes
- Pension plans
- Unemployment compensation
- Worker's compensation
- Life and disability
- Hospital insurance
- Medical services
- Tuition reimbursement
- Vacation pay
- Holiday pay
- Sick leave

Each of these benefits should be budgeted on the basis of the terms of the benefit—the amount, the positions covered, and any limitations. Benefit expenses are typically spread according to the timing of the actual expense. Those expenses that relate directly to the dollar amount of salaries and wages can be spread as a percentage of salary expense. Depending on the terms, some benefit expenditures are fixed in nature, and others flex directly with payroll expenditures.

Chapter 13

Supplies, Purchased Services, and Other Expenses Budget

I n budgeting for supplies, purchased services, and other expenses, it is important to determine the relationship of these expenses to units of service. If the expense varies with changes in volume, that relationship must be considered in preparing the budget. If the expense within a natural category is variable, the general methodology for budgeting the expense is to accumulate and analyze information about current expenditures on a per unit basis, adjust the per unit value for inflation and known or anticipated changes, and multiply the adjusted per unit value by the budgeted units of service. If the expense varies in step levels, the calculation is adjusted to determine different values for each of the levels of service up to and beyond the budgeted level. Although cumbersome, this level-by-level calculation is helpful in analyzing variances during the budget year.

Supplies Expenses

The changes in supplies expenses from year to year are primarily the result of volume and price changes; substitution has a minor impact. Volume requirements of supplies and other expenses are more closely related to changes in the amount of services rendered than are salaries and wages.

Volume depends on several factors. Increased supply volume, for example, may be caused by an increased number of patients receiving the same services, the same number of patients receiving more tests or more procedures (intensity), or a different mix of patients receiving more procedures or a different set of procedures (change in mix as a result of new programs). It is important to be able to analyze budget estimates from line managers in terms of volume and price; to relate projected changes in patient days, patient mix, or types of service to projected changes in supply volume; and to relate price projections to past experience and unpublished indexes.

The relationship between supply volume and patient services is particularly important for departments that offer services directly to patients, for example, food service, central service, and laboratory. Changes in patient services have less effect on indirect services, such as maintenance and housekeeping. Both maintenance and housekeeping services usually remain relatively constant whether the nursing units are 88 percent or 78 percent occupied.

Supply and other expenses must be budgeted in the month they are actually used in order to match expenses with patient service revenue. Statistics are again important.

Statistics provide the means to allocate the individual expense to particular months and to evaluate the reasonableness of some expense estimates on an overall basis. Food service costs, for example, vary with the number of patients served, and so it would be appropriate to allocate the food cost by month on the basis of budgeted patient days. On the other hand, housekeeping costs may be related to changes in the number of square feet from period to period.

The definition of individual expense categories is important in obtaining consistent projections from line managers. The budget package sent to line managers for their completion should include descriptions of items that would be properly included in each expense category. The following examples are based on adaptations of the natural classification of expenses system suggested by the American Hospital Association in its *Chart of Accounts for Hospitals* (Chicago: American Hospital Publishing, 1976):

> *Laboratory supplies* – includes the cost of all laboratory supplies, for example, cells, culture media, chemicals, glassware, forceps, dressing, reagents, tubing, pipettes, stainless steel utensils, micro slides, filter paper, cover glasses, flasks, test tubes, and drugs ordered by the laboratories for their use.
> *Medical and surgical supplies* – includes the cost of all medical and surgical supplies ordered by departments other than the laboratory, for example, identification bands, adhesive, bandages, blades and brushes, catheters, surgeon's gloves, hypodermic needles, suture needles, sutures of all types, splints, crutches, and so forth.
> *Housekeeping supplies* – includes the cost of all cleaning and housekeeping supplies, for example, brooms, brushes, mops, dustpans, garbage cans, polish, waxes, insecticides, disinfectants, deodorants, detergents, toilet tissue, soaps used for other than laundry purposes, and so forth.
> *Laundry supplies* – includes the cost of all laundry supplies, for example, soaps, bleaches, asbestos pads, covers, dyes, and so forth.
> *General maintenance supplies* – includes the cost of all general maintenance supplies, for example, casters, bolts, nuts, screws, lubricants, small tools, welding gases, solder, rods, and so forth.

Each of these natural classifications relates to one or another of the supply classifications shown in the operating budget. Additional special classifications not shown would include disposable linen, radioactive materials, and supplies charged to patients. The nature and specificity of the account depend on the needs of the hospital.

Supply expenses can be estimated in a variety of ways for budgeting purposes. Any method used should include comparisons of volume and unit cost budgeted and comparable statistics from actual experience. One method for determining reasonableness that can also be used for controlling costs in the budget period is to request that the appropriate line manager list the 20 supply items that cost the most together with an indication of the volume and the projected unit cost. A sample work sheet for this type of analysis is shown in figure 13-1. The month-by-month analysis for the current and budget years is helpful for isolating and explaining trends and specific variances. The list of the largest purchases is helpful for control during the budget year in that it provides a basis for comparing actual volume and unit cost for individual items to budgeted cost.

By using actual patient days and medical supply costs from prior years, medical and surgical supplies expenses for one department may be estimated for the budget year by using a work sheet similar to the one shown in figure 13-2. Once the total amount of supply expense has been estimated, it should be allocated to the months of the budget year on the basis of patient days, as shown in figure 13-3.

In figure 13-2, all medical and surgical supplies are included in the same classification, and so it is necessary to have each line manager estimate the medical and surgical supply expense. The total expense for the hospital should not be related only

Figure 13-1. Work Sheet for Analyzing Monthly Expenses for Largest Individual Purchases

General Hospital
Expense Work Sheet (Supplies)—Budget 1992

Department No.: _____   Department Description: _____
Expense Account No.: _____   Account Description: _____   Date: _____
Prepared by: _____

Actual/ Projected 1991	1992 Budget	List of Largest Individual Items to Be Purchased			
		Description	Quantity	Unit Price	Extension
		1.		$	$
		2.			
		3.			
Jan. $____	$____	4.			
Feb. ____	____	5.			
March ____	____	6.			
April ____	____	7.			
May ____	____	8.			
June ____	____	9.			
July ____	____	10.			
Aug. ____	____	11.			
Sept. ____	____	12.			
Oct. ____	____	13.			
Nov. ____	____	14.			
Dec. ____	____	15.			
		16.			
Total $____	$____	17.			
		18.			
		19.			
		20.			

Total Items Listed $_____
Total Other Items $_____
Total Budget $_____

to patient days because the expense category includes operating room and emergency department supplies that relate more closely to the use of the operating room or to emergency department visits.

Other supply costs, such as patient food costs, can be related directly to patient days for volume changes. Film expenses can be related to the number of procedures in diagnostic radiology. Pharmacy expenses relate primarily to patient days but may also include the use of pharmaceutical supplies in the operating room (fluids) and the emergency department. In the case of the pharmacy, the line manager may want to analyze the volume and unit cost changes as shown for medical and surgical supplies in figure 13-2 and, in addition, list the 20 items that cost the most as shown in figure 13-1, for subsequent variance analysis.

Purchased Services Expenses

Purchased services include such items as commissions and fees, utilities, rentals, professional services, service contracts, and telephone service. One way to estimate purchased services is to list the major expected expenditures by month for each of the purchased services accounts and compare them to the actual projected figures for the current year and, possibly, to the actual expenditure for the prior year. The format used should allow for comparison by month and provide ample space for explaining variances.

The line manager compares the individual items on the list with the prior year's list and with the list of projected expenses from the current year's budget for variance analysis. This type of listing is also helpful for control purposes during the year. An example of a simple work sheet for this comparison is shown in figure 13-4. This

---

Figure 13-2. Work Sheet for Estimating Medical and Surgical Supplies Expenses for an Intensive Care Unit

General Hospital
Estimate of Medical and Surgical Supplies—1992 Budget

Department: NURSING—INTENSIVE CARE UNIT 121   Prepared by: _____

Year	Patient Days	Medical and Surgical Supplies Cost	Average Cost per Day	Percent Increase Average Cost
1989	3,250	$56,712	$17.45	5.5
1990	2,935	54,620	18.61	6.7
1991	3,000	59,850	19.95	7.2

1991 average cost per day	$19.95
1992 estimated price increase (10.5%)	×1.105
1992 estimated average cost per day	$22.04
1992 estimated patient days for ICU	×3,009
1992 estimated medical and surgical supply cost for ICU	$66,330

Figure 13-3. Monthly Allocation of Medical and Surgical Supplies Expenses for an Intensive Care Unit

General Hospital
Monthly Allocation of Medical and Surgical Supplies—1992 Budget

Department: NURSING—INTENSIVE CARE UNIT 121   Prepared by: _____

Month	Budget Patient Days	Budget Medical and Surgical Supplies
January	246	$ 5,424
February	236	5,204
March	241	5,314
April	251	5,535
May	261	5,755
June	251	5,535
July	251	5,535
August	260	5,733
September	260	5,733
October	250	5,512
November	261	5,755
December	241	5,313
Total	3,009	$66,348

Figure 13-4. Work Sheet for Comparing Purchased Services Expenses for Past, Current, and Budget Years

General Hospital
Expense Work Sheet (Purchased Services)—1992 Budget

Department No.: _____
Expense
Account No.: _____

Account
Description: _____

Department Description: _____

Prepared by: _____   Date: _____

Description of Individual Service	Jan.	Feb.	March	April	May	June	July	Aug.	Sept.	Oct.	Nov.	Dec.	Total
1992 budgeted monthly total													
1991 projected monthly total													
1990 actual monthly total													

Explanation of variances: _____

work sheet may be used for purchased services that are contracted by individual line managers for their responsibility centers (commissions and fees, rentals, and professional services) as well as by managers with overall responsibilities (utilities, service contracts, and telephone service).

Other Expenses

The remaining portion of the expense budget includes items such as travel and association dues that are budgeted in individual responsibility centers and items such as interest, depreciation, and insurance that apply to the whole institution and are budgeted separately. For both types of expenses, an acceptable technique is to base the monthly estimate on historical trends of actual monthly expenditures for the current and prior years and adjust these figures for known changes in service, hospital policy, and anticipated prices. Estimates for travel, meeting expense, and association dues are prepared by line managers who should be able to explain the rationale for each month's estimate. Interest projections can be calculated from existing and anticipated outstanding debt. Depreciation can be calculated from lapsing schedules or similar property records and adjusted for completion of building or renovation and installation of new equipment. Insurance is estimated with the help of the insurance broker when the insurance premium period does not correspond with the fiscal year or with an actuary when the hospital is self-insured.

Completed Expense Budget

The completed expense budget has a separate budget for each responsibility center. Each responsibility center budget shows budgeted monthly expenditures and statistics.

Figure 13-5. Monthly Operating Expense Budget for an Intensive Care Unit

General Hospital
Operating Expense Budget—1992 Budget

		Month/Intensive Care Patient Days[a]				
Number	Account Description	Jan./246	Feb./236	March/241	April/251	May/261
6121.01	Registered nurse	$18,775	$16,973	$18,775	$18,255	$18,810
6121.02	Nurse assistant	698	630	698	675	698
6121.03	Licensed practical nurse	2,533	2,284	2,533	2,453	2,566
6121.04	Ward clerk	2,103	1,903	2,103	2,102	2,103
6121.06	Head nurse	3,926	3,591	3,926	3,800	3,926
6121.36	Medical and surgical supplies	5,437	5,202	5,321	5,533	5,752
6121.37	Drugs (floor stock)	1,311	1,254	1,283	1,334	1,387
6121.38	Disposable linen	294	282	289	300	312
6121.46	Office and administrative supplies	49	47	48	50	52
6121.49	Minor equipment	202	196	201	209	217
6121.50	Other supplies	147	141	144	150	156
6121.56	Equipment repairs and maintenance	180	174	176	183	191
6121.77	Equipment rental	268	257	263	274	284
		$35,923	$32,934	$35,760	$35,318	$36,454

[a]Use ancillary procedures or other statistics instead of patient days when appropriate. Purpose is to give reviewer a description of the level of activity.

The estimates are approved by the appropriate line managers before they are submitted to the budget director for consolidation. The review and approval of the appropriate line managers is indicated by their signatures on the budgets.

The completed expense budget may be submitted in the format shown in figure 13-5, which shows the monthly expense budget for an intensive care unit. This responsibility center, along with all other responsibility centers, has to be consolidated along functional classifications for inclusion in the overall operating budget summaries. This consolidation results in a functional subgrouping for registered nurses' salaries and wages, which in turn is a part of total salaries and wages.

Similar analyses are performed for all other nursing classifications. The sum total of the several nursing classifications would represent the total salaries and wages for nursing personnel. Performing these classification groupings permits analysis and comparison (year to year for the hospital or to other hospitals or to industry standards) of similar costs by function. Depending on the organization of the hospital, this level of classification detail may be necessary to allow reporting and control along the established lines of responsibility within the organization. The totals by job category broken down into their fixed and variable components would be the basic reporting categories for productivity reports prepared each pay period and included in the monthly flex-budget reports.

The full expense budget that has now been analyzed by responsibility unit and by function is submitted to the budget committee for review. No final decisions can be made at this point in the budget cycle because the budget committee has only established general revenue policies and reviewed the operating statistics. What the committee now has in hand are the projected costs of operating at the level defined by the statistics. The committee has not seen the projections for patient revenue, allowances, and other revenue, nor has it seen the cash budget, capital budget, or projected balance sheet.

Figure 13-5. (Continued)

Responsibility Unit: 121   Description: Intensive Care Unit
Prepared by: _____   Approved by: _____

Month/Intensive Care Patient Days[a]

June/251	July/251	Aug./201	Sept./260	Oct./250	Nov./261	Dec./241	Total 3,009	1991 Projection 3,000
$18,378	$18,982	$19,091	$18,516	$19,093	$18,483	$19,092	$223,223	
675	725	698	675	698	675	698	8,243	
2,486	2,533	2,577	2,453	2,533	2,453	2,533	29,937	
2,036	2,130	2,103	2,036	2,103	2,036	2,103	24,861	
3,839	3,926	3,926	3,850	3,926	3,800	3,926	46,362	
5,533	5,533	5,732	5,732	5,514	5,752	5,314	66,355	
1,334	1,334	1,382	1,382	1,330	1,387	1,282	16,000	
300	300	312	312	299	312	288	3,600	
50	50	52	52	50	52	48	600	
209	209	216	216	208	217	200	2,500	
150	150	156	156	150	156	144	1,800	
183	183	190	190	183	191	176	2,200	
274	274	283	283	273	284	263	3,280	
$35,447	$36,329	$36,718	$35,853	$36,360	$35,798	$36,067	$428,961	

Chapter 14

Cash Budget

The objectives of cash planning are the following:
- To have sufficient cash to meet maturing debt obligations
- To maintain a cash flow sufficient to replace and/or expand hospital facilities in accordance with long-term plans for meeting the needs of the community
- To have sufficient cash to meet anticipated working capital requirements and a reasonable contingency to cover unanticipated requirements
- To establish a prudent program for the investment of cash in excess of current requirements

The basic document for cash planning is a detailed cash budget. This document summarizes cash receipts and cash disbursements for regular intervals, usually each month, during the budget year and projects cash balances at the end of each interval. The cash budget includes the following:
- Cash receipts from operations
- Cash disbursements from operations
- Nonoperating cash receipts and disbursements
- Summary document

The cash budget is developed and finalized simultaneously with the capital budget and before the projected balance sheets are prepared. The first attempt at a cash budget is a learning experience. Once the cash budget has been used for a year, the subsequent years' budgets will provide more refined estimates with less effort.

Cash Receipts from Operations

The largest item of cash receipts is the collection of accounts receivable. When cash receipts are budgeted the payment policies of the various types of payers, such as Medicare, Medicaid, other state or local programs, Blue Cross, commercial insurance companies, health maintenance organizations, and self-pay patients, must be considered. Anticipated economic conditions, the previous history of each payer, and the payer's payment mechanism are the major elements in anticipating collection.

Most payers recognize the obligation and make the payment after the service is performed and a bill is submitted that meets their requirements. A few payers still use a periodic interim payment mechanism whereby the hospital receives a regular payment based on budgeted utilization. A quarterly adjustment is usually performed to bring the payments up-to-date. At year end, a reconciliation is performed and a final settlement is made to complete payment for services during the year.

Medicare pays hospitals for services to covered patients on the basis of the diagnosis-related group (DRG) into which the patient falls. The DRG payment covers most of Medicare's contractual obligation. A cost report filed at the end of each year contains the final adjustments and calculations of the amount due to or due from Medicare to close out the amount to be received for services provided to Medicare patients.

The traditional Medicaid payment system provides payment for actual services on the basis of a calculated per diem rate or percentage of charges. This system also provides a settlement payment after a year-end reconciliation pertaining to actual costs. Other government payment programs depend on local regulation and availability of funds.

Payment systems for Blue Cross plans and other commercial insurance plans vary. Some may pay on the basis of negotiated charges, a discount from charges, or a per diem or per case amount. Specific contract requirements may identify certification or length-of-stay limitations for certain types of cases. Health maintenance organizations and payers with similar contracts may also pay a specified monthly capitation for specific services for all individuals enrolled in a special plan.

The presence of an overall state rate authority may affect any or all of these payment mechanisms and may introduce additional variables, such as discounts for prompt payments or penalties for late payments.

The hospital's overall collection experience can be determined by reviewing a sequential aging analysis of accounts receivable for a single month's billing. For example, a review of the January 1992 billings that remain in the accounts receivable balance at the end of February, March, April, and May can be the basis for calculating the percentage collected in the periods following the month of service (0 to 30 days, 31 to 60 days, 61 to 90 days) and ultimately the general collectibility of the January billings. These percentage factors can be used to project the timing of cash collection of future billings. Figure 14-1 presents such an analysis for four months of accounts to be collected. Collection experience analysis as described is most useful for charge-based payers. A separate analysis should be prepared for payers that use interim payment plans.

Current interim payment amounts can be adjusted to the anticipated level at the beginning of the budget year and then calculated for each month of the budget year on the basis of budgeted monthly expenditures and projected changes in utilization. There are four steps in this overall analysis:

Figure 14-1. Analysis of Collection of Accounts Receivable Balance

General Hospital
Analysis of Patient Accounts Receivable—Beginning of Budget Year 1992

Month of Billing	Amount Remaining to Be Collected	Month of Collection			
		Jan.	Feb.	March	April
September	$ 268,000	$ 268,000	$	$	$
October	421,000	281,000	140,000		
November	926,000	463,000	308,000	155,000	
December	1,625,000	813,000	406,000	271,000	135,000
Total	$3,240,000	$1,825,000	$854,000	$426,000	$135,000

- The timing for the collection of existing accounts receivable at the beginning of the budget year is estimated by using the aging analysis procedure just described (shown in figure 14-1).
- The net amount to be billed each payer each month is determined. As shown in figure 14-2, this is done by projecting the net patient revenue by month from the monthly gross patient revenue and deductions from revenue. The cash that will be collected from outpatients at the time of service and/or deposits from inpatients on admission are taken into consideration when the amounts are significant.
- Cash receipts from operations are estimated by month. Figure 14-3 illustrates the collection of the accounts receivable balance at the beginning of the year and the conversion of net billed revenue into estimated cash receipts by month. The analysis also shows the total amount of receivables collected during the year. The uncollected amount represents the net accounts receivable that would appear on a balance sheet projected for the end of the budget year. The cash collections from outpatients are derived from the analysis of the projected monthly net revenue billed (figure 14-2) and are shown as a separate item after the net revenues billed for patient services.
- Receipts from other operating and nonoperating revenue are estimates. The monthly collections are based on historical experience in most cases and include some or all of the following:
  - Nursing school tuition is probably collected at the beginning of each quarter or semester.
  - Endowment fund earnings, which may be restricted for a special purpose such as free care or nursing school tuition, are shown in the analysis for the period when the special purpose expenditures are expected to be made. When the funds are unrestricted, they appear in the analysis for the budget period when the earnings will be available for operating use.
  - Cafeteria and parking income is shown when it is collected. Both of these functions are cash-basis operations for income, but their expenses are treated like the expenses from any other cost center.

Figure 14-2.   Analysis of Net Patient Revenue to Be Billed by Month

General Hospital

Projected Monthly Net Revenue Billed for Budget Year 1992

Month	Gross Revenue Patient Services	Deductions from Revenue	Net Revenue for Patient Services	Cash Collected from Outpatients	Monthly Net Revenue Billed
January	$ 1,948,210	$ 188,244	$ 1,759,966	$ 21,000	$ 1,738,966
February	1,855,440	179,280	1,676,160	21,000	1,655,160
March	2,087,370	201,690	1,885,680	21,000	1,864,680
April	1,948,210	188,244	1,759,966	21,000	1,738,966
May	2,087,370	201,690	1,885,680	21,000	1,864,680
June	1,994,590	192,725	1,801,865	21,000	1,780,865
July	1,994,590	192,725	1,801,865	21,000	1,780,865
August	1,762,670	170,316	1,592,354	21,000	1,571,354
September	1,855,440	179,280	1,676,160	21,000	1,655,160
October	1,948,210	188,244	1,759,966	21,000	1,738,966
November	1,855,440	179,280	1,676,160	21,000	1,655,160
December	1,855,460	179,282	1,676,178	21,000	1,655,178
Total	$23,193,000	$2,241,000	$20,952,000	$252,000	$20,700,000

— Sales revenues from snack shops and gift shops run by the institution's aux- iliary are budgeted on the basis of historical experience and discussions with the auxiliary about the timing and the amounts of revenue transfers to the hospital. If the snack shop and gift shop are run by the hospital, the income is recorded when collected, and the expenses are recorded just as the expenses for any other cost center are recorded.

Significant nonoperating cash receipts are not included with the operating receipts. Rather, they are shown as a separate line item or line items on the cash receipts and disbursements summary (figure 14-3).

If its first attempts at estimating cash collections result in unrealistic estimates, the hospital should reexamine its previous experience. A cash analysis of the actual experience during the past two years can be performed with consideration of monthly gross revenue versus net revenue billed, month of collection, and other income amounts. Unusual receipts or disbursements in prior periods should also be identified. These might include large third-party settlements or cash delays caused by implementation of a new billing system, which should be excluded from the percentages used in prepar- ing the cash budget. When in doubt, it is better to underestimate than to overestimate cash collection.

Figure 14-3. Cash Receipts Summary

General Hospital
Analysis of Cash Receipts for Budget Year 1992

Patient Receivables	Net Patient Receivables to Be Collected	Jan.	Feb.	March	April	May	June
Beginning balance	$ 3,240,000	$1,825,000	$ 854,000	$ 426,000	$ 135,000	$	$
January	1,739,000		869,500	434,750	295,630	139,120	
February	1,655,000			827,500	413,750	281,350	132,400
March	1,865,000				932,500	481,250	327,050
April	1,739,000					894,500	459,750
May	1,865,000						957,500
June	1,781,000						
July	1,781,000						
August	1,571,000						
September	1,655,000						
October	1,739,000						
November	1,655,000						
December	1,655,000						
Net revenue	$20,700,000	$1,825,000	$1,723,500	$1,688,250	$1,776,880	$1,796,220	$1,876,700
Subtotals	$23,940,000	$1,825,000	$1,723,500	$1,688,250	$1,776,880	$1,796,220	$1,876,700
Other cash collections:							
Outpatient services		$ 21,000	$ 21,000	$ 21,000	$ 21,000	$ 21,000	$ 21,000
Gift shop		12,000	11,500	12,800	12,300	12,800	12,300
Cafeteria		12,300	11,100	12,400	12,100	12,400	12,100
Other nonpatient care revenue	$ 130,000	25,000	22,000	21,000	22,000	22,000	21,000
Subtotals		$ 70,300	$ 65,600	$ 67,200	$ 67,400	$ 68,200	$ 66,400
Estimated cash receipts from operations		$1,895,300	$1,789,100	$1,755,450	$1,844,280	$1,864,420	$1,943,100

Cash Disbursements from Operations

The two major disbursements for operations are:
- Payroll
- Supplies and other expenses

Payroll, the most significant disbursement, usually accounts for more than 60 percent of total expenditures. Whereas the expense budget considers wages earned, the cash budget considers only the wages paid. Therefore, the monthly payroll expenses must be translated to disbursements on a cash basis.

Most hospital employees are paid biweekly (every two weeks); however, some are paid semimonthly or monthly. Because payday is usually several days after the end of the pay period, paydays seldom coincide with the end of the month or fiscal year. Therefore, in converting an expense budget to a cash budget, accruals and the actual date of payment must be considered at the beginning and end of each period. Also to be considered is the fact that some months have two biweekly paydays and some have three.

The source for the payroll disbursement projections is usually the same as that used for the payroll expense budget. This source is the personnel budget. An example of a format for converting monthly payroll expense to monthly cash disbursements

Figure 14-3.   (Continued)

July	Aug.	Sept.	Oct.	Nov.	Dec.	Total Cash Collected	Uncollected Net Patient Receivables
$	$	$	$	$	$	$ 3,240,000	$
						1,739,000	
						1,655,000	
124,200						1,865,000	
270,630	114,120					1,739,000	
441,250	292,050	124,200	50,000			1,865,000	
865,500	420,250	277,770	167,480	50,000		1,781,000	
	865,500	420,250	327,770	167,480		1,781,100	
		735,500	392,750	292,070	100,680	1,521,000	50,000
			802,500	413,750	181,350	1,397,600	257,400
				844,500	323,400	1,167,900	571,100
					527,500	527,500	1,127,500
							1,655,000
$1,701,580	$1,691,920	$1,557,720	$1,740,500	$1,767,800	$1,132,930	$20,279,000	$3,661,000
$1,701,580	$1,691,920	$1,557,720	$1,740,500	$1,767,800	$1,132,930	$20,279,000	$3,661,000
$ 21,000	$ 21,000	$ 21,000	$ 21,000	$ 21,000	$ 21,000	$ 252,000	$
12,700	12,800	12,300	12,700	12,300	13,500	150,000	
12,400	12,400	12,100	12,400	12,000	12,300	146,000	
22,000	22,000	22,000	21,000	21,000	21,000	262,000	$ 100,000
$ 68,100		$ 68,200	$ 67,400	$ 67,100	$ 66,300	$ 67,800	$ 810,000
$1,769,680	$1,760,120	$1,625,120	$1,807,600	$1,834,100	$1,200,730	$21,089,000	

appears in figure 14-4. The months with three pay periods, the recognition of the delay from the end of the pay period to the date of payment (time required to prepare and distribute pay), and the accruals at the beginning and end of the budget year should be noted. The accrual at the end of the budget year should be part of the total accrued liability on a projected balance sheet for that date.

Payroll taxes and fringe benefits appear in the cash budget as an item separate from salary and wages because the timing of most tax payments is different than the pay date. Furthermore, tax payments represent a payment in addition to gross payroll.

Calculations of Social Security taxes in the expense budget are helpful in computing the payroll deduction for these taxes. Because the hospital matches the

Figure 14-4. Sample Format for Converting Monthly Payroll Expense to Monthly Cash Disbursements

General Hospital
Analysis of Monthly Salary and Wage Disbursements for Budget Year 1992

Month	Budget Expense	Pay Period Ending Biweekly	Pay Period Ending Monthly	Gross Payroll Biweekly	Gross Payroll Monthly	Total Gross Monthly Disbursement
January	$ 837,300	12/28/91 01/11/92 01/25/92	01/31/92	$362,000 362,000 356,000	$ 40,000	$ 1,120,000
February	755,900	02/08/92 02/22/92	02/28/92	358,000 358,000	40,000	756,000
March	846,100	03/08/92 03/22/92	03/31/92	364,000 364,000	40,000	768,000
April	824,800	04/05/92 04/19/92	04/30/92	366,000 366,000	40,000	772,000
May	863,700	05/03/92 05/17/92	05/31/92	374,000 374,000	40,000	788,000
June	841,400	05/30/92 06/14/92	06/30/92	374,000 374,000	40,000	788,000
July	890,200	06/28/92 07/12/92 07/26/92	07/31/92	384,000 384,000 384,000	40,000	1,192,000
August	899,000	08/09/92 08/23/92	08/31/92	388,000 388,000	40,000	816,000
September	875,800	09/06/92 09/20/92	09/30/92	390,000 390,000	40,000	820,000
October	916,600	10/04/92 10/18/92	10/31/92	396,000 396,000	40,000	832,000
November	892,800	11/01/92 11/15/92	11/30/92	398,000 398,000	40,000	836,000
December	925,400	11/29/92 12/13/92 12/27/92	12/31/92	400,000 400,000	40,000	840,000
Total budget expense	$10,369,000	Total cash disbursements for salary and wages				$10,328,000
		Accrued 12/31/92				(458,000)
		Accrued 12/31/92				499,000
		Total budget expenses				$10,369,000

employees' contributions, the percentages used in the expense calculation can also be used for the payroll deduction calculation.

Calculations of income tax withholding are based on historical experience and recent revisions in the tax laws. The only reason for listing this amount separately is to indicate the different timing for the disbursement of payroll and payroll taxes.

Deductions from salary for other fringe benefits, such as for parking privileges, may require no cash disbursement. Other deductions, such as health insurance coverage for dependents, will require a separate payment even though they are not institutional expenses.

Estimates of the amount of the payroll deduction and the timing of payment are made on the basis of past experience. In analyses of cash disbursements (figure 14-5), employer taxes are included with fringe benefits and are shown as a separate line item. When the timing of the payment of taxes is significantly different from the monthly payroll, the format shown in figure 14-6 can be used for the payroll analysis.

Physician fees representing payments to such groups as radiologists, pathologists, and cardiologists are also shown as a separate line on the cash analysis when they are on a separate line in the expense budget.

Supplies and other expenses are broken down for estimating cash disbursements. Basically, supplies and other expenses fall into two separate disbursement groups: those that require regular monthly purchases, such as medical supplies and office supplies, and those that require irregular disbursements, such as premiums on professional liability insurance, interest, and audit fees.

Medical and office supplies can be estimated on the basis of historical payments. Adjustments are required for the inventory at the beginning and end of the year. Medical supplies, office supplies, and all other regularly scheduled payments may also be projected by using an analysis of accounts payable similar to the accounts receivable analysis.

As shown in figure 14-5, other significant disbursements, such as interest on long-term debt, premiums for professional liability insurance and other types of insurance, supplies and other regularly scheduled expenses, and audit fees, are shown separately on the disbursement schedule. Each of these expenses represents an irregular payment, which requires a separate projection of cash requirements.

Nonoperating Cash Receipts and Disbursements

Cash receipts and disbursements analyzed to this point have been related only to operations. However, the cash flow of a hospital includes sources of, and requirements for, cash other than operations. Sources of cash other than operations include:

- Investment income, which should be based on an analysis of the hospital's portfolio
- Sale of investments, which is made on the basis of cash requirements and known maturities
- Gifts for capital, which are estimated on the basis of the historical experience of the development office
- Sale of assets, which are based on an analysis of replacement items in the capital budget

Requirements for cash other than operations might include:

- Principal payments, calculated from an analysis of debt contracts
- Equipment purchases, indicated in the capital budget (chapter 15)
- Building renovation or expansion, also indicated in the capital budget or by special capital analysis
- Purchase of investments, based on an analysis of cash requirements

Figure 14-5. Analysis of Cash Disbursements

General Hospital

Analysis of Cash Disbursements for Operations for Budget Year 1992

Description	Totals	Jan.	Feb.	March	April
Salaries and wages	$10,328,000	$1,120,000	$ 756,000	$ 768,000	$ 772,000
Fringe benefits	1,351,000	147,259	99,974	101,325	102,676
Supplies and other regularly scheduled expenses	6,500,000	526,500	546,000	520,000	585,000
Audit fees[a]	30,000		5,000	10,000	5,000
Professional liability and other insurance[b]	603,000	302,000		151,000	
Interest, net of interest income	256,000			64,000	
Estimated disbursements for operations	$19,068,000	$2,095,759	$1,406,974	$1,614,325	$1,464,676

[a]Audit fees include payments for completion of 1991 audit and preliminary work on the 1992 audit.

[b]Premium year in this example is calendar year.

Summary Document

A cash receipts and disbursements summary analysis is prepared in order to anticipate the hospital's cash position on a month-to-month basis throughout the budget year. A format for a cash receipt and disbursement summary is shown in figure 14-7. The document shows summary information for each month and distinguishes between operating and nonoperating sources of, and requirements for, cash. During the year, a more detailed schedule based on actual experience and expected changes is used for analyzing investment opportunities. Long-term forecasts that show the cash receipts and disbursements for the next three to five years in less detail should also be prepared and updated annually. A narrative description of significant assumptions should accompany both the budgeted cash receipts and disbursements summary and a long-range cash forecast.

The gain or loss resulting from changes in the market value of restricted assets is a noncash item that is reflected in the analysis of change in fund balance. It does not, however, affect the cash receipts and disbursements summary.

The transfer between funds, such as the transfer between the operating fund and the plant fund (when a plant fund is maintained in the accounts), is usually a bookkeeping transfer only. It does not affect the cash receipts and disbursements summary.

Projecting cash receipts and disbursements on a monthly basis facilitates the planning of investments or temporary borrowing decisions and thus optimizes the use of cash. During the budget period, cash forecasts showing estimates of cash receipts and disbursements on a daily basis for a week or two in advance should be prepared for management. Longer-term (usually five-year) projections are frequently prepared in connection with debt financing to determine the ability of the hospital to meet the payment schedule for the requested debt. The same process may be used to prepare the long-term forecast. However, because of the nature of the projection, the description and the related amounts of the various types of cash receipts and disbursements should be summarized, and annual amounts should be shown in lieu of monthly estimates.

If management found it desirable to analyze the transactions in a special fund, an investment account, or a pool of investments, the format that appears in figure 14-5 might be used. Analyzing all sources of cash is helpful in planning and coordinating the optimum utilization of all available funds.

Figure 14-5. (Continued)

	May	June	July	Aug.	Sept.	Oct.	Nov.	Dec.
	$ 788,000	$ 788,000	$1,192,000	$ 816,000	$ 820,000	$ 832,000	$ 836,000	$ 840,000
	104,027	104,027	158,067	106,729	108,080	108,080	106,729	104,027
	546,000	578,500	552,500	552,500	487,500	526,500	552,500	526,500
						5,000	5,000	
	150,000							
		64,000			64,000			64,000
	$1,588,027	$1,534,527	$1,902,567	$1,475,229	$1,479,580	$1,471,580	$1,500,229	$1,534,527

Figure 14-6. Analysis of Payroll Disbursements When Taxes and Payroll Payment Timing Differ

General Hospital

Analysis of Payroll Disbursements for Budget Year 1992

Month	Monthly Payment	Less Taxes Withheld		Other Deductions	Net Pay for Salary and Wages
		Income	Social Security		
January	$ 1,120,000	$ 172,480	$ 66,416	$ 14,660	$ 866,444
February	756,000	116,424	44,982	14,660	579,934
March	768,000	118,272	45,850	14,660	589,218
April	772,000	118,888	46,010	14,660	592,442
May	788,000	121,352	46,965	14,660	605,023
June	788,000	121,352	47,044	14,660	604,944
July	1,192,000	183,568	71,162	14,660	922,610
August	816,000	125,664	48,307	14,660	627,369
September	820,000	126,280	48,544	14,660	630,516
October	832,000	128,128	48,672	14,660	640,540
November	836,000	128,744	48,237	14,660	644,359
December	840,000	129,360	46,956	14,660	649,024
Total	$10,328,000	$1,590,512	$609,145	$175,920	$7,952,423

Figure 14-7. Summary Analysis of Cash Receipts and Disbursements by Month

General Hospital
Cash Receipts and Disbursements Summary for Budget Year 1992

Receipts and Disbursements	Jan.	Feb.	March	April	May	June
Beginning balance—cash and investments	$ 300,000	$ 26,291	$ 226,117	$ 218,792	$ 405,896	$ 559,789
Add: receipts from operations	1,895,300	1,789,100	1,755,450	1,844,280	1,864,420	1,943,100
Less: disbursements for operations	2,095,759	1,406,974	1,614,325	1,464,676	1,588,027	1,534,527
	$ 99,541	$ 408,417	$ 367,242	$ 598,396	$ 682,289	$ 968,362
Other nonoperating cash receipts (disbursements):						
Payment on long-term debt	—		(54,000)			(54,000)
Purchase of capital assets	(73,250)	(82,300)	(94,450)	(92,500)	(72,500)	(93,000)
Transfer to "funds designated for future expansion"	—	(100,000)	—	(100,000)	(50,000)	(50,000)
Ending balance—cash and investments	$ 26,291	$ 226,117	$ 218,792	$ 405,896	$ 559,789	$ 771,362

Figure 14-7. (Continued)

July	Aug.	Sept.	Oct.	Nov.	Dec.	Total
$ 771,362	$ 522,175	$ 652,666	$ 608,906	$ 807,926	$1,035,597	$ 300,000
1,769,680	1,760,120	1,625,120	1,807,600	1,834,100	1,200,730	21,089,000
1,902,567	1,475,229	1,479,580	1,471,580	1,500,229	1,534,527	19,068,000
$ 638,475	$ 807,066	$ 798,206	$ 944,926	$1,141,797	$ 701,800	$ 2,321,000
		(54,000)			(53,000)	(215,000)
(66,300)	(104,400)	(85,300)	(87,000)	(56,200)	(108,800)	(1,016,000)
(50,000)	(50,000)	(50,000)	(50,000)	(50,000)	(40,000)	(590,000)
$ 522,175	$ 652,666	$ 608,906	$ 807,926	$1,035,597	$ 500,000	$ 500,000

Chapter 15

Capital Budget

Which comes first, the cash budget or the capital budget? Each depends on the other, and so clearly the two should be prepared at the same time. The cash budget must provide the amount of cash required to purchase capital, and the capital budget must have the amount of cash available to purchase capital items. Because more capital items are usually requested than can be purchased with available funds, cash availability should be determined by the time capital requests are assigned priorities. The consolidation of information from these two budgets takes place toward the end of the budget process, and both are included in the same operating budget package for review by the governing board.

The capital budget is a plan that identifies the major asset items that have been assigned a high priority for purchase and the expected source of funds required to make the purchase. Figure 15-1 presents a simple flowchart showing the steps usually required to complete a capital budget.

Capital budgeting involves strategic planning. Well-planned capital decisions are needed to attain the long-range goals of the hospital. The capital budget is part of the operating budget and reflects planned expenditures for at least a three-year period. A three-year capital plan makes good business sense and is required by Medicare's Conditions of Participation. Some hospital managers may even prepare a capital budget that covers five years. In either case, the capital budget should not be a wish-list with every requested item included. Doing so fails to communicate priorities, does not recognize limited resources to purchase capital, and leads to disappointment and unmet expectations among department and clinical managers.

Sources of capital vary but in general include hospital resources resulting from operating income, debt (including leases), funded depreciation, unrestricted investments, proceeds from the sale of assets, and endowment income; federal, state, and local assistance in the form of grants and contracts; and philanthropy (gifts, bequests, and proceeds from organized fund drives). These sources are used for new and replacement equipment and for facility improvement. Borrowed funds backed by mortgages or pledges of revenue currently supply the largest portion of resources for major capital projects (facilities, expansion, or replacement). In developing the estimate of cash availability, it is necessary to project operating results and philanthropy in order to analyze the availability of unrestricted investments and the need and availability of borrowed funds.

Figure 15-1. Flowchart of Capital Budget Process

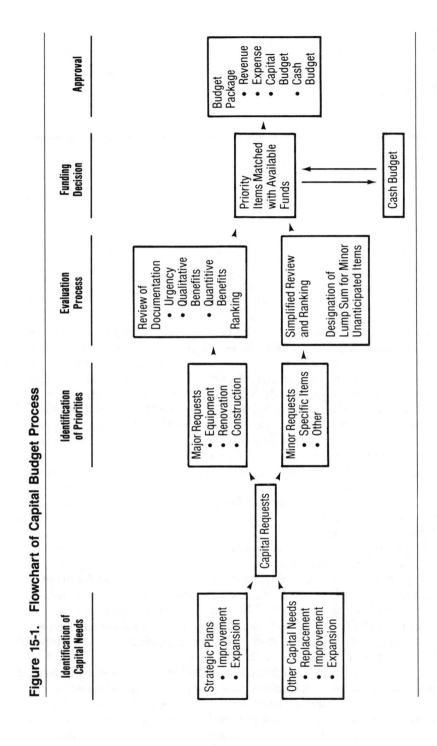

The capital budget usually includes expenditures for anticipated major construction, renovation, or repairs; proposed acquisitions of equipment to facilitate expansion of existing services or addition of new services to keep up with current technology; and replacement of current plant and equipment at prices that reflect inflation and current technology. The capital budget also provides for an amount of undesignated dollars for contingencies, emergency capital equipment replacements, and discretionary activity on the part of administration. This amount, although minor, permits additional purchases without disrupting planned purchases or requiring lengthy studies and reassignment of priorities. Under provisions of federal planning legislation, capital acquisitions that cost more than a prescribed amount or that provide new services must be subjected to a lengthy public approval process. The time requirements, and sometimes the documentation or review criteria, should be considered when scheduling the purchase of major items. Of course, repairs, even major repairs, that do not increase the value of an asset or extend its useful life are expense items in the operating budget, are not capitalized on the balance sheet, and are not a part of the capital budget process.

Capital Expenditure Requests

Capital expenditure requests originate at the department level, where line managers working with appropriate clinical staff can identify needs for the coming year, justify each request, and make an initial determination of priorities within their areas of responsibility. It is also important that an organized process for the internal review of capital expenditures exists. Requests and priority ranking developed by each department manager and appropriate medical staff should be reviewed and discussed with the managers of all other affected departments before being submitted to the budget committee. Careful planning is required, and managers must be reminded not to commit themselves without specific budget approval. Although inclusion in the budget does not constitute authorization to purchase, usually only those expenditures approved in the planning process are made during the budget year.

During the budget process and even after the budget has been approved, it is often necessary to remind every individual involved that the capital budget is a forecast of capital requests to purchase the items, not an approval. Sometimes, especially when the review process is thorough, individuals believe that the decision to purchase has been made and forget that, as the budget fiscal year unfolds, priorities may change or funds may not be available as planned.

Funding for capital projects is limited by the hospital's ability to generate capital. The sources of capital are few. The primary source is the operating margin plus certain noncash expenditures, such as depreciation. The availability of capital funds from debt, which is really a mortgage on future income, also depends on the hospital's ability to generate net income. Interestingly, the development of funds from philanthropy is also made easier when the hospital has a proven ability to generate net income.

It is the responsibility of management to provide a formal approval process and the criteria for project evaluation. The approval process should differentiate between minor and major projects. Requests for items that require a small expenditure should be accompanied by less documentation to justify the project than would requests for large expenditures. An explanation of what constitutes major and minor expenditures is made by management and included in the instructions distributed to line managers. For example, the hospital president may approve expenditures (assuming that funds are available) for minor items costing less than a specified amount, say $10,000. On the basis of this guideline, items that cost more than the specified amount, $10,000 and above, must have the approval of the governing board. Of course, all items that cost more than the regulatory minimum or that will provide a new service must also go through the certificate-of-need process.

Each request should indicate the month or quarter of the budget year during which the expenditure is to be made. This is needed to develop an accurate cash disbursement estimate for the cash budget and for longer-term cash projections.

Each department's priority list is reviewed by the purchasing department or the controller's office to verify the purchase price. Large projects are reviewed by construction experts before being approved for inclusion in the capital budget so that surprises in price and time requirements are eliminated. Often, a request is made for purchase of equipment long before the equipment could be installed, even if it were ordered at the time the request was submitted. The delay may be caused by the need to modify facilities prior to installation or by custom equipment fabrication requirements.

Evaluation criteria or justification may be expressed by indicating the necessity of the request and by answering a series of questions. The degree of necessity may be expressed in one of the following ways:

- Urgent
- Essential
- Economically desirable
- Generally desirable

Following are examples of questions that should be answered if the request is marked urgent, essential, or economically desirable:

- *Safety:* Does the present situation present a hazard to patients? To employees? Have there been specific incidents?
- *Agency requirements:* Is this request in response to the requirement of an outside agency, such as the Joint Commission on Accreditation of Healthcare Organizations? How else might the requirement be met? Is a less costly solution equally satisfactory? Does this request meet the code requirements of appropriate agencies (for example, United Laboratories)?
- *Patient care:* How will this item improve patient care?
- *Equipment replacement:* Is this the only piece of equipment that performs this function in the department, or is it one of several? How crucial is it to the department's operation? Are maintenance costs excessive compared with replacement costs? Does unreliable performance create extra work load or cause unsatisfactory results?
- *Revenue producing:* How much and what kind of new revenue will the new project produce?
- *Cost reduction:* How will spending funds on this item reduce overall expenditures? Will it increase productivity?

Obviously, if a sense of urgency were the only criterion for funding capital projects, department managers would be encouraged to overstate current deficiencies, and choosing projects for funding would be based on eliminating current deficiencies rather than on building toward longer-term positive improvements. Therefore, every request should answer the following questions:

- If a request represents a new service, why is the service necessary?
- If it is a service expansion:
  - Will the expenditure result in an increase in the volume of procedures?
  - Where is the demand for these procedures?
  - Is the capacity of existing equipment inadequate, or could additional labor hours expand the service as economically and as appropriately as could providing new capital?

- If the request represents a service improvement:
  - How is the quality of the current service deficient, and will the proposed expenditure remedy this deficiency?
  - How will the proposed expenditure make a good service better?
- Regardless of whether the request represents a new service, service expansion, or service improvement:
  - Will this request require additional space to locate the capital item or supporting staff?
  - Will the proposed expenditure increase or decrease labor costs in the requesting department or other centers?
  - What will be the cost of supplies and maintenance?
  - What other means of meeting the need were considered? Why were they rejected?
  - What action would have to be taken if the request were not funded?

Basically, the commonsense rule is to encourage the department manager to anticipate the questions that will be asked by senior management and, to the degree possible, respond to those anticipated questions in the request. It will make the process of establishing priorities go more smoothly and, from the department manager's viewpoint, will increase the possibility of having the requests reviewed favorably.

Some requests lend themselves to quantitative analysis. The decision to make or buy an item may be expressed in the relative costs and benefits of either option. The decision to commit to a capital expenditure may be based on a comparison of the cost of instituting a new service, continuing a current service, or improving the service with the cost of contracting for the same service from an outside vendor or joining with other organizations to develop a shared service. Individual revenue-producing or cost-saving requests should be analyzed in terms of payback or rate of return. If quantitative techniques could provide better information for the evaluation process, they should be incorporated into the formal project evaluation. However, the instructions provided to the person doing the analysis should emphasize that the various methods of quantitative analysis are only tools to assist administration in making a sound decision. Qualitative factors are frequently as important or sometimes even more important than quantitative factors. Whatever evaluation techniques are employed, it is important to institute and use some formal criteria to evaluate capital requests so that limited resources are used effectively. The form shown in figure 15-2 may be used by a single department to request minor capital equipment expenditures.

Because not all requests for minor capital items can be anticipated, it may be necessary to provide an undesignated amount to be used for other minor capital items at the discretion of the president. If such an amount is required, it should be included in the capital budget along with any restrictions on its use (that is, the funds can only be used for unanticipated minor capital expenditures approved by the president).

Major items should be summarized on a single form in order of priority by a department manager. The same form might also be used to highlight important justifications for the purchase. A form that may be adopted for that purpose is shown in figure 15-3. Because major items are usually requested for the next three years, a separate list should be prepared for each year.

Supporting each priority list should be a document that provides the answers to all the previously indicated questions and any other information that is pertinent to each item on the list. Of course, the information is expected to be more complete for those items requested for the first year than for those requested for the second or third year. A simple listing of items with comments may be sufficient for the second and third years. A single-page form may be useful as a summary for each request and also as a checklist of the information to be included in the documentation for use by the responsibility center manager. Such a form appears in figure 15-4.

Figure 15-2. Sample Form for Requesting Minor Capital Equipment Expenditures

General Hospital
Minor Capital Equipment Request for Budget Year 19____   Page ____ of ____

Department no. _____   Description: _____

Department manager: _____   Extension: _____

Itemize below, in order of priority, proposed capital expenditures having a useful life of one year or more and costing $500 to $XXXX.

Description	Cost per Unit	Number of Units	Total Cost	Month Required	New equipment	Generally desirable	Economically desirable	Essential	Urgent
						(✓) Where Appropriate			

Figure 15-3. Sample Form for Listing Major Capital Equipment Expenditures Requested by a Department

General Hospital

Summary of Capital Equipment Requested   Page _____ of _____

For budget year 19____

Department no. _____   Description _____

Approvals: Department manager: _____
           Medical staff _____
           Financial manager _____

Itemize below, in order of priority, all proposed capital expenditures having a useful life of one year or more and costing $_____ to $_____.

Item #	Description	Amount	Comments

Figure 15-4. Sample Form for Summarizing Capital Equipment Expenditure Requested Information for One Item

General Hospital   Item no._____

Capital Request Work Sheet for Budget Year 19____   Page_____ of _____

Department no. _____   Description_____

Approvals: Department manager: _____
            Medical staff _____
            Financial manager _____
            (purchase price verification)

Description of item _____

Cost per unit $_____ Number of units_____ Total cost _____

Month/year to be ordered_____ Month/year required _____

New service/expansion/improvement _____

Estimated new annual revenue/cost saving _____

Urgent/essential/desirable _____

Space/FTE requirement _____

(Reason for requesting item: please respond fully to information requested above)

The larger the request, the more documentation required. For major requests, a more comprehensive work sheet or checklist should be developed to ensure that all information required for evaluation is provided by the department manager. Again, the definition of a major capital expenditure is to be determined by those responsible for selecting the projects to be funded.

Final Preparations

It is at the point at which the budget committee establishes priorities for the requests and makes funding decisions that the capital budget and the cash budget come together. Depending on the nature of the requests, the cash generated from the operating budget (budgeted net income plus the noncash expenditures such as depreciation and amortization) is usually sufficient to cover the purchase of minor, new, and replacement equipment and to build up resources for major, new, or replacement capital projects. Because the matching of resources available for capital and capital requests is shown in the cash budget, both the approval of the capital budget and the finalization of the cash budget must be completed at the same time. Estimates of available resources are derived from the operating budget, current balance sheet, an analysis of debt availability, and occasionally the revenue-producing ability of the capital items themselves.

After estimates of available resources and responsibility center requests for capital acquisitions have been made, a final listing of selected projects can be prepared for the governing board's approval. Once again, the final process of selecting what capital expenditures will be made is a joint effort and should include input from the department managers and medical staff as well as the president and other members of the budget committee. During the selection process, the lists submitted by the department managers may well be revised as the managers and medical staff see what has been included or excluded from the list. When the final list is prepared for the governing board, it should be accompanied by a schedule that shows the source of cash to be made available for the contemplated purchases (cash budget). A summary of the justification supplied by the department manager and appropriate comments from the president for some items on the list can also be given to the governing board.

The sample format that appears in figure 15-5 can be used for listing capital expenditures for inclusion in the operating budget package. A sample capital budget is

Figure 15-5. Sample Form for Listing All Capital Equipment Expenditures

General Hospital
Capital Budget for Year 19_____

Department/Item Description	Month of Purchase	Estimated Payment			
		First Quarter	Second Quarter	Third Quarter	Fourth Quarter

included in the model operating budget in the appendix. Only a few departments are shown in the sample listing; however, every major item and a total for the minor items should be included in a complete, final list. This list shows the month of purchase, full amount of the expenditures, and estimated quarter of payment. For some projects, it may be appropriate to schedule the payments by month. Although a list such as the one that appears in the appendix should include all capital building, remodeling, and renovation items in detail, a separate report with additional information can be prepared for the governing board if the capital budget is to include major facility expansion or new construction.

When the capital budget is complete, information from it is included in the cash budget and that document finalized for review by the governing board as part of the total budget package. In the model operating budget in the appendix, the statement on changes in financial position shows that enough cash is available from operations to pay for the capital budget items.

In another period or in another institution, funds from philanthropy may be available. It may be necessary to sell investments or incur indebtedness to get the necessary cash to purchase the required capital.

The preparation of the capital budget usually involves the allocation of scarce resources to a variety of projects, and the amount of capital requested in the initial department listings will usually exceed the resources available. If the organization is to grow in an orderly fashion, specific procedures for evaluating the requests and matching them to available resources are essential.

The actual determination of funded projects is guided by the goals and objectives expressed in the hospital's long-range plan and is the result of line management, senior management, and the medical staff working together. Because the estimation of available resources is a standard part of the cash budget and the cash budget must include the capital requirements, both budgets are developed and approved simultaneously.

Chapter 16

Balance Sheet

At this point in the budgeting process, projections have been completed for operating revenue and expenses, cash, accounts receivable, and capital transactions. A stack of work sheets showing calculations and assumptions supports each of the budget schedules. To determine the impact of the successful implementation of the proposed budget on the hospital's financial position, a balance sheet should be prepared that projects the hospital's financial position at the end of the budget year.

The balance sheet summarizes in one page the work done in the preceding steps. It shows what management thinks the financial position of the hospital will be at the end of the year if all assumptions are accurate and if operations closely match the budget. It serves as a focal point for pulling together many of the budget decisions and formulates some of the planned results in terms of goals for managing assets during the budget year. To be meaningful, therefore, the operating budget should include a balance sheet that compares the projected balances at the end of the current fiscal year to the balances projected at the end of the budget year, along with a narrative describing the assumptions that were used in developing the balance sheet.

In addition to being used in projections of the hospital's financial position at the end of the budget year, the schedules and assumptions are used by senior management and the governing board to formulate goals for the management of hospital assets, particularly cash and accounts receivable. The work sheets that support the cash receipts analysis will contain a number of calculations that were made to project a reasonable level of collections. The number of days in accounts receivable at the end of each month in the budget year, based on the expected revenue and collections, should have been calculated and compared with the actual experience in prior years. Although prepared as a test of the reasonableness of anticipated collections, the calculations also provide monthly balances of projected patient services receivables for comparison to the actual results during the budget year.

Similarly, the number of days in accounts payable may have been calculated when the cash disbursement schedule was prepared. This type of calculation will be useful in establishing a standard against which to evaluate the accounts payable balances, as compared with the budget, through the budget year.

In some instances, the assumptions made earlier in the budget process will provide a basis for calculating the projected balances but will not provide the balances themselves. The amount due from Medicare and Medicaid is the result of many factors, including program utilization and changing regulations. The interim payment rate assumptions made in connection with work done on the analysis of cash receipts will be helpful in projecting a balance due (or payable to) Medicare and Medicaid at the end of the budget year.

Sources of Figures

In the projected balance sheet shown in figure 16-1, many of the balances come directly from schedules shown in previous chapters. Some balances can be calculated on the

Figure 16-1. Balance Sheet

General Hospital
Balance Sheet—Projected 1991 and Budget 1992

Assets	Projected 1991	Budget 1992
Current assets		
Cash and investments	$ 300,000	$ 500,000
Patient services receivables, net of allowances of $360,000 in 1991 and $407,000 in 1992	3,240,000	3,661,000
Due from Medicare and Medicaid	177,000	177,000
Other accounts receivable	130,000	100,000
Other current assets	414,000	490,000
Total current assets	$ 4,261,000	$ 4,928,000
Property and equipment		
Land and buildings	$14,594,000	$14,620,000
Movable equipment	4,156,000	5,006,000
Construction in process	106,000	246,000
	$18,856,000	$19,872,000
Less accumulated depreciation	(5,250,000)	(6,322,000)
Total property and equipment	$13,606,000	$13,550,000
Funds designated for future expansion	$ 1,668,000	$ 2,258,000
Endowment and other restricted investments	$ 1,340,000	$ 1,360,000
Total assets	$20,875,000	$22,096,000

Liabilities and Fund Balances	Projected 1991	Budget 1992
Current liabilities		
Accounts payable	$ 300,000	$ 500,000
Salaries, wages, and other accruals	460,000	680,000
Portion of long-term debt due within one year	215,000	255,000
Total current liabilities	$ 975,000	$ 1,435,000
Long-term debt, less current portion	$ 2,900,000	$ 2,645,000
Fund balances		
Unrestricted funds	$15,660,000	$16,656,000
Endowment and other restricted funds	1,340,000	1,360,000
Total fund balances	$17,000,000	$18,016,000
Total liabilities and fund balances	$20,875,000	$22,096,000

basis of work done on other budget schedules, and other balances relate only generally to those schedules. In particular:

- Cash and investments are taken directly from the cash receipts and disbursements summary.
- Patient services receivables and other accounts receivables balances are taken directly from the analysis of cash receipts.
- The amount due from Medicare and Medicaid is estimated by considering projected cost increases, interim payments, program utilization, and projected settlements of open years.
- Other current assets are projected on the basis of an analysis of the items included in this category. The items in the analysis are projected to the end of the current year and to the end of the budget year.
- Property and equipment changes are based on the capital budget and projected retirement of major items.
- Increases in funds designated for future expansion are taken directly from the cash receipts and disbursement summary.
- Endowment and other restricted investments balances change only because of the projected receipt of restricted gifts or use of the funds in accordance with donors' restrictions.
- Accounts payable is estimated on the basis of a recent analysis of vendor disbursement days in accounts payable. For purposes of this calculation, a vendor disbursement day equals the amount paid during the recent year for supplies and other regularly scheduled expenses divided by 365. The product is then divided into the accounts payable balance for the end of the prior year to determine the vendor disbursement days in accounts payable. The cash disbursements for supplies and other regularly scheduled expenses shown in the analysis of cash disbursements is divided by 365. The product is multiplied by the current vendor disbursement days in accounts payable to project a balance to the end of the budget year. Some simple ratios of accounts payable to cash disbursements result in a similar projection.
- Salaries, wages, and other accruals are based on the analysis of monthly salary and wage disbursements plus an analysis of other accounts in this category.
- Long-term debt and the portion of long-term debt due within one year are taken from payment schedules that are part of the loan agreements.
- Unrestricted funds increase only because of changes in budgeted net income. When more activity is expected, a separate analysis of changes in the unrestricted fund balance should accompany the projected balance sheet.
- Endowment and other restricted funds increase only as a result of contributions projected during the budget year or the use of funds in accordance with donors' restrictions. When significant transactions are expected in this classification, a separate analysis of changes in the fund balance should accompany the projected balance sheet.

The amount of detail expressed in a forecasted balance sheet and the sophistication of the estimates or the analysis depend on the significance of the amounts and the intended use of the balance sheet. Because the forecasted balance sheet is the result of so many estimates and assumptions, detail tends to be misleading. General or overall calculations are sufficient for estimating immaterial amounts.

Once the balance sheet has been prepared for the budget year and the assumptions have been written, new balance sheets and operating, cash, and capital budgets can be prepared for several additional years. A few additional assumptions are made, and the balance is projected forward.

Change in Financial Position

When the projected balance sheet is complete, the next step is the completion of a statement of change in financial position for the budget year. The most useful format is the reconciliation of cash balance from the beginning of the budget year to the end, as the changes show in the financial position report of the model operating budget. (See the appendix.) In this format, the statement summarizes the cash budget and focuses on the changes in the balance sheet that require further discussion and analysis. Once the revenue and expense budgets and the capital and cash budgets have been completed, the preparation of the projected balance sheet and statement of changes in financial position is relatively easy because the projected statements are summary statements that focus on changes in the hospital's financial position from the beginning of the budget year to the end.

Chapter 17

Operating Reports

When all the schedules have been completed and the operating budget prepared, there should still be time for an overall review of the final product. Is it complete? Are all variances explained? Are all calculations correct? Most important, is the budget reasonable, and does it properly reflect management's operating plan? If so, the final operating budget is ready to go to the budget committee and then to the governing board for its approval. At this point in the process, it is important to review the operating reports that will be used to compare actual results to budget during the coming year.

In chapters 2 and 3, the need for a systematic method of management reporting and accountability at all levels was discussed. During the budget process, statistics and performance measures were developed at the operating department level, the clinical department level, and the program level. The statistics were converted to dollar amounts, which were then consolidated to form the hospital's budget.

It is now necessary to incorporate the budget information into the control system. The budget director must go back to the source documents, identify the statistics and other performance measures that were adopted for use in the budget, and incorporate these into the management reporting system. To be effective tools for management control, the reports must be timely. In some cases, they must reflect daily comparisons of actual performance and budget performance and, in other cases, weekly, biweekly, or monthly comparisons. The reports must also provide a basis for analyzing variances both in statistics and in dollar amounts.

Because this book has emphasized the flexible budgeting concepts, units of service are used to project statistics and develop budgeted revenue and expense. Therefore, when the budget is finalized and the control mechanism (namely, the management reporting system) is updated, these statistics should be included in the operating reports for all levels of management. When statistics are included on the reports, the department manager, budget director, and senior management can compare performance to budget in terms of volume and expense. For example, if a department's volume and expenses were twice the budgeted amount, comparing the center's performance to the fixed budget would show a significant unfavorable variance. If the units of service, both budget and actual, and the fixed and variable characteristics of the cost were utilized in a flexed report, the amount expended could easily be compared with the expected expenditure, as adjusted for actual volumes. The nature of the variance is made much more clear, and the information is more useful for control purposes.

Daily Reports

Daily reports should be provided for cash, patient revenue, and census. Because department-level statistics are developed on a monthly basis, those statistics must be broken down to a daily basis. There is a limit, however, to the amount of detail that can be projected and reasonably used for control purposes. Is it worthwhile, for example, to budget a daily census for each nursing unit, or is it just as useful to compare each day's census to the budgeted average for the month? Should a daily cash balance be predicted? Perhaps only the actual daily cash balances should be reported, and cash flow from patients (or specific payer groups) should be compared for the day and/or month to date, prior months in the same year, or similar periods in prior years (adjusted for rate increases). Daily accounts receivables balances by major payer category are also helpful in establishing trends and focusing on significant change. The forms in figures 17-1, 17-2, 17-3, and 17-4 can be used for reporting information at the beginning of each day. These suggested reports are certainly not a complete set of daily reports but are a few examples that managers might find helpful. Additional reports may be required to analyze progress in troublesome areas. In accounts receivable, for example, it may be advisable to monitor, in more detail, the movement of accounts through the process to better identify those areas requiring quick attention.

The report in figure 17-4 requires additional preparation because each month's budgeted occupancy must be broken down by day of the month, with weekends and holidays taken into consideration. The additional effort is clearly worthwhile because it allows management to tell at a glance how well daily operations compare to budget. The variance may be analyzed in terms of the average per diem charge variance and the occupancy variance. In the example in figure 17-4, the $11,567 favorable variance can be analyzed as follows (differences are the result of rounding off to the nearest penny):

Per diem variance

= (actual per diem − budget per diem) × actual days

= {[$420,641 actual inpatient revenue ÷ (7 days × 215 actual average occupancy)] − [$409,074 budget inpatient revenue ÷ (7 days × 214 budget average occupancy)]}

(7 × 215)

= ($279.50 − 273.08) × 1,505

= $9,662 better than budget

Occupancy variance

= (actual occupancy − budget occupancy) × budget per diem

= [(97 × 215) − (7 × 214)] × $273.08

= (1,505 − 1,498) × $273.08

= $1,912 better than budget

Figure 17-1. Sample Format for Daily Cash Report

General Hospital

Daily Cash Report   Date: _____

Distribution: _____

		Daily Transactions			
Description	**Beginning Balance**	**Deposits**[a]	**Disbursements**[b]	**Ending Balance**
Cash accounts:				
First Bank general account				
First Bank special account				
National Bank payroll "A"				
National Bank payroll "B"				
Security deposits				
Hospital working capital funds				
Total cash				
Short-term investments				
Short-term (CDs)				
First Bank special account				
Total investment short-term				
Total cash and investments				

Ending Balance Prior Month

Deposits	**Daily**	**Month to Date**
Cash[c]		
S.N.F. checks		
Notice of credit		
Voided checks		
Investment income		
Transfers from other accounts		
Total		

General Account Activity

Disbursements	**Daily**	**Month to date**
Vendor payments		
Special payments ("quick pays")		
Payroll disbursements		
Advice of debit		
State taxes		
Federal taxes		
Total		

[a]Total daily deposits from the General Account Activity form.
[b]Total daily disbursements from the General Account Activity form.
[c]Daily cash deposit ties to total on the comparative statement of monthly cash collections report (figure 17-2).

157

Figure 17-2. Sample Format for Report of Comparisons of Cash Collections by Month

General Hospital
Comparative Statement—Cash Collection
Receipts through _____ (Working days _____)

Distribution: _____

Type of Deposit	Daily Deposits	Current Month to Date	Prior Months—Same Working Days (or same date)				
			(Nov.)	(Oct.)	(Sept.)	(Aug.)	(July)
Inpatient:							
Commercial insurance							
State agency—cash							
Medicare—cash							
Blue Cross—cash							
Patient payment							
Outpatient:							
Patient payment							
Commercial insurance							
State agency							
Medicare							
Blue Cross							
Total patient receivables collected							
Other deposits							
Less cash transfers to other accounts	( )	( )	( )	( )	( )	( )	( )
Total cash deposit to general account[a]							

[a]Total ties to daily cash deposit on Daily Cash Report.

Figure 17-3. Sample Format for Reporting Receivables

General Hospital   Distribution: _____
Analysis of Accounts Receivables
Date: _____

| | | Patient Days in Accounts Receivable | |
		Actual	Budget
Unbilled accounts			
In-house	$ _____	_____	_____
Recent discharges (normal hold)	_____	_____	_____
Late[a]	_____	_____	_____
Total unbilled accounts	$ _____	_____	_____
Billed accounts			
Patient			
Commercial insurance			
State agency			
Medicare			
Blue Cross	_____	_____	_____
Total billed accounts	$ _____	_____	_____
Other			
Unmatched inpatient charges			
Unmatched inpatient cash	(_____)	(_____)	(_____)
Total other	$ _____	_____	_____
Total inpatient accounts receivable	$ _____	_____	_____
Total outpatient accounts receivable	$ _____	_____	_____
Total accounts receivable	$ _____	_____	_____
Average revenue per patient day	$ _____	_____	_____

[a]Late includes accounts held for diagnosis or pending acceptance for state medical aid program.

Figure 17-4. Sample Format for Comparing Actual Daily Inpatient Revenue to Budget for One Month

General Hospital   Distribution: _____
Daily Inpatient Revenue Report
Comparison of Actual to Budget for December 1991

| Days Revenue | Average Occupancy Month to Date | | Revenue Month to Date | | Better (Worse) than Budget |
	Budget	Actual	Budget	Actual	
1 (Mon.)	219	211	$ 59,804	$ 57,953	($ 1,851)
2	219	217	119,609	125,667	6,058
3	220	221	180,232	190,135	9,903
4	220	221	240,310	249,107	8,707
5	217	218	296,292	306,036	9,744
6 (Sat.)	214	215	350,635	361,126	10,491
7 (Sun.)	214	215	409,074	420,641	11,567
8	215		469,698		
9	217		533,325		
10	218		595,314		

Weekly Reports

Knowing the daily cash balance is helpful, but having a good estimate of the weekly cash balance is even more helpful. Cash projections made in the cash budget help plan the sources and uses of cash during the year, when all goes according to the budget. The budget cannot predict all events, and so it is reasonable to expect that the cash projections will have to be constantly updated. One type of projection is a longer-term, perhaps three-month, projection that is updated monthly. This should preclude any major surprises related to unexpected cash requirements. In terms of daily cash management, it is also helpful to have a weekly forecast prepared at the beginning of each week that projects the sources and uses of cash for the remainder of the week. The weekly forecast will help prioritize payments and facilitate the use of a line of credit, if necessary.

Biweekly (Payroll) Reports

The reports in figures 17-5 and 17-6 could be prepared and distributed after each payroll cycle. A variation of the report in figure 17-5 could be prepared to summarize the data for the year to date. Payroll expense is the largest single item on the income statement. Personnel is the largest single hospital resource. Personnel cost must be monitored frequently at the department level and at the consolidated hospital level. The use of a statistic such as the paid full-time equivalent (FTE) per equivalent occupied bed enables management to review the appropriateness of the staffing as the number of hours paid changes to meet the needs of increasing or decreasing patient service volumes. (Equivalent occupied bed refers to a statistic developed by adjusting the census to reflect an equivalent amount of outpatient services.) At the department level, the detailed data by position (job code) (see figure 17-6) shows the breakdown of the hours and the dollars paid for regular time, overtime, vacation, holiday, and sick time.

Monthly Reports

Monthly reports can be prepared in a variety of formats and are variable in terms of historical period shown. The daily reports that have month-to-date amounts or that show the balances as of the last day of the month (such as those shown in figures 17-1, 17-2, and 17-4) are the first indicators of the month's results. The next report to be issued at month end might be a summary of key indicators of the month's activity prepared from data gathered at month end or from a preliminary close of certain accounts that are not expected to change in the final close. A typical key indicator report might compare the following information to budget for the month and for the year to date:

- Activity:
  - Admissions
  - Patient days (adult)
  - Average length of stay
  - Average daily census
  - Percent occupancy (operational beds)
- Payer mix percentage (by patient days):
  - Medicare
  - Medicaid
  - Commercial insurance

Figure 17-5. Sample Format for a Full-Time Equivalent (FTE) Summary

General Hospital
Full-Time Equivalent (FTE) Summary
Period covered—through March 8, 1991

Pay Period End Date	Paid Man-Hours[a]	Full-Time Equivalent (FTE)			Overtime (OT)		Average 2-Week Equivalent Census	FTE per Equivalent Occupied Bed (EOB)		
		Paid FTE	Budget FTE	Favorable (Unfavorable)	Overtime Man-Hours	Overtime Hours/Total Man-Hours		Paid FTE/EOB	Budget FTE/EOB	Favorable (Unfavorable)
Jan. 11	59,459	743	733	(10)	1,903	.032	220	3.38	3.15	(.23)
Jan. 25	56,806	710	733	23	1,250	.022	224	3.17	3.15	(.02)
Feb. 8	57,022	713	733	20	1,312	.023	227	3.14	3.15	.01
Feb. 22	5,283	741	733	(7)	1,423	.024	236	3.14	3.15	.01
Mar. 8	59,786	747	733	(14)	1,315	.022	238	3.14	3.15	.01

[a]Excludes paid hours covered by grants or research funds.

Figure 17-6. Sample Format for a Labor FTE Report—Department Summary

General Hospital
Labor FTE Report—Department Summary
Department—Intensive Care Unit
Department Number—121
Pay Period End Date—March 8, 1991

Cost Center	Code	Position Title	Regular Hours	Overtime Hours	VHS[a] Hours	Total Hours	Paid FTE	Budget FTE	Regular Dollars	Overtime Dollars	VHS[a] Dollars	Total Dollars
121	01	Registered nurse	1,148	32	48	1,228	15.35	16.00	$11,675	$488	$488	$12,651
121	02	Nurse assistant	72	—	8	80	1.00	1.00	585	—	65	650
121	03	Licensed practical nurse	160	27	—	187	2.34	3.00	1,370	347	—	1,717
121	04	Ward clerk	240	—	—	240	3.00	3.00	1,673	—	—	1,673
121	06	Head nurse	240	18	8	266	3.33	3.00	2,791	314	93	3,198
			1,860	77	64	2,001	25.02	26.00	$18,094	$1,149	$646	$19,889

[a]VHS stands for vacation, holiday, and sick time.

- Health maintenance organization/preferred provider organization
- Self-pay/other
- Salaries:
  - Wages paid
  - Overtime hours as a percentage of total hours
  - FTE paid (nonfunded)
  - FTE per equivalent occupied bed
- Cash and marketable securities
- Patient accounts receivable:
  - Total patient accounts receivable
  - Average days outstanding
  - Cash collected
- Accounts payable:
  - Unpaid invoices
  - Cash disbursed

Certain of these information items might also be trended or graphed for the past six months to show trends and historical variance from budget.

Full reports prepared after the monthly closing come later in the monthly reporting cycle. They have, however, more detailed comparisons for the revenue and expense budget, balance sheet, cash budget, and capital budget.

Monthly reports provide management with two types of information:
- Revenue and expense comparisons and capital expenditure comparisons by department or cost center (these reports should show statistics as well as dollar amounts)
- Revenue and expense account comparisons at various levels from functional groups down to departments or cost centers (functional reports)

A department budget is developed along established organizational lines. In figure 3-2, at least four separate levels of responsibility were easily identified. The basic unit is a cost center or group of cost centers (a department or responsibility center) with a person responsible (a line manager).

The governing board and senior management establish the long-term goals of the institution. Together with senior management, the line managers develop the operating plan. The line managers also prepare the detailed budgets for implementing the operating plan. The reporting system should provide information to line managers that enables them to take necessary corrective actions and control the areas for which they are responsible. The greatest amount of management information detail should be available at the line-manager level. Just as the authority of the more senior levels of management is broader, the information presented at these levels tends to include summaries of the detailed data available to line managers. Reports to the governing board provide comparisons for the hospital as a whole and resemble the format of the consolidated financial statements in the model operating budget. Reports for senior management and the governing board should be accompanied by concise explanations covering what happened and why. The explanations should not include basic calculations, such as how much a particular item was over budget, especially when the variance is already shown in the report.

A line-management report for a nursing intensive care unit might use a form such as the one shown in figure 17-7. The form does not include allocated or indirect expenses; rather, it focuses on the expenses that the line manager is reasonably expected to control. The patient days and the revenue are included on the report for comparative purposes. The combined nursing service responsibility report for the appropriate senior manager would reflect the results of all nursing units in a format that includes only the total expenses for each nursing unit.

Figure 17-7. Sample Format for Department Budget Comparison

General Hospital
Department Budget Comparison—March 1991
Department—Nursing Intensive Care Unit
Department Number—121

Current Month					Year to Date			
Budget	Actual	Flexed Budget	Variance		Budget	Actual	Flexed Budget	Variance
═══	═══	═══	═══	Total patient days	═══	═══	═══	═══
				Revenue:				
───	───	───	───	Patient room charge	───	───	───	───
───	───	───	───	Other patient charges	───	───	───	───
═══	═══	═══	═══	Total revenue	═══	═══	═══	═══
				Wages and salary expense:				
───	───	───	───	Wages	───	───	───	───
───	───	───	───	Overtime	───	───	───	───
═══	═══	═══	═══	Total wages	═══	═══	═══	═══
				Other expenses:				
───	───	───	───	Medical/surgical supplies	───	───	───	───
───	───	───	───	Drugs	───	───	───	───
───	───	───	───	Disposable linen	───	───	───	───
───	───	───	───	Office and administrative supplies	───	───	───	───
───	───	───	───	Minor equipment	───	───	───	───
───	───	───	───	Other supplies	───	───	───	───
───	───	───	───	Equipment repairs and maintenance	───	───	───	───
───	───	───	───	Equipment rental	───	───	───	───
═══	═══	═══	═══	Total other expenses	═══	═══	═══	═══
═══	═══	═══	═══	Total expenses	═══	═══	═══	═══

A report for an ancillary department would be similar in format, but the descriptions would vary to reflect the differences in the nature and significance of the revenue and expense items. For example, revenue for a laboratory might be classified into at least two categories to reflect inpatient and outpatient test revenue. When units are indicated on each report at the responsibility-center level, it is possible to analyze the variances in terms of unit values. Examples of this type of analysis, which show the impact of both cost and volume factors, were discussed in previous chapters.

The daily basic revenue (room charges) and ancillary revenue should be supported by a number of comparative reports. Given that it is assumed that the daily basic charge schedules vary little during the year, basic daily revenue for inpatients is a function of patient days. Patient days are budgeted for each service by the administrative staff together with the medical staff (chapter 11). Patient-day comparisons that show patient days or occupancy percentages or both should be included in a routine monthly report.

Ancillary revenue was estimated on the basis of monthly statistics for each department. Those statistics, reflecting the actual volume of services as compared to budget, should also be a routine monthly report. The relative value units used to price the ancillary tests can be used by management to evaluate the change in volume in constant terms. When possible, line managers should be provided with comparative reports for each service provided and billed by their responsibility centers.

Personnel statistics deserve special attention in the budget process, and they deserve special attention in the management reports as well. Presumably, line managers know the staffing of each of their responsibility centers; however, they should have available and utilize reports such as those discussed in chapter 5, which help analyze the effectiveness of the personnel in relation to the actual volume of services. It is more difficult for senior managers to keep track of total staffing than it is for line managers, and for that reason it is worthwhile to prepare separate routine monthly reports showing actual staffing by job classification compared with budgeted staffing levels flexed for actual activity levels.

Generally, line managers should be provided with comparative information in the same detail that was requested for the budget. The reporting process should require that line managers use these reports to explain significant variances between actual and budgeted activity and highlight potential future problems for senior management. The significance of variance should be determined by the person receiving the information (senior management). Often, it is expressed in terms of a percentage, but because small amounts tend to vary by large percentages, it is preferable to define significance for reporting in terms of a percentage *and* a minimum dollar amount.

Whereas most of the traditional reports are department based, the up-to-date reporting package should also include program analyses comparing actual to budget revenues and expenses and statistics for general program categories and for specific programs. Program results as compared to operating objectives should be discussed in the operating reports. It is at this level that senior management and the board can determine the hospital's progress toward strategic goals and relate improvements in patient service and the attainment of specific program goals with the resources required to attain those goals.

Significant variations should be explained by the department or program manager on an ongoing and timely basis. The variance explanations should be carried forward, as appropriate, to the monthly financial statement package that is prepared for senior management and the governing board.

The overall financial position of the hospital is the responsibility of senior management, particularly the chief executive officer, and the governing board. Evaluation of the financial position is best facilitated by comparison of actual to budgeted results in a form similar to that used in the operating budget. A typical package for facilitating this process should include a revenue and expense comparison (similar to the format of income and expenses report for the model operating budget in the appendix) but including a column showing the flexed budget expenses. Statistical highlights and explanations of significant variances should accompany the comparison. Supporting the revenue and expense comparison might be a comparison of occupancy statistics (similar to the information contained in the occupancy statistics report for the model operating budget in the appendix) and a comparison of the average per diem and per procedure charges (similar to the information contained in the model operating budget). All revenue and expense schedules should show comparative amounts and statistics for the most recent month and the year to date. Simple charts are very effective in reflecting trends. The package should also include a balance sheet comparing the most current month to the prior month and/or to the balance at the beginning of the fiscal year, a statement of changes in financial position for the month and year to date, and statements of changes in fund balances for the month and the year to date. A summary of the aging of accounts receivable by major payer category would also be a useful report to include in the package. The governing board may also be interested in one or more special reports, such as an analysis of the investments at cost and market value as of month end and, during a major construction project, an analysis of the construction activity.

Because every hospital board is different and board members have their preferences, the contents of the reporting package should be determined by the board. Some board members are happy with charts showing summary variance and trends. Others want to know exactly what is happening with accounts receivable. The reports should be tailored to provide the information requested. For example, a board member who manages his or her own business might want information similar to what is used to manage his or her business's operations. The person may use a daily report that includes the cash balance, the backlog, the accounts receivable over 60 days, and the total accounts payable. If those statistics were in order each day, he or she might not have to look for any further detail. For this type of person, a summary statement of revenue and expense and the key indicator statistics, discussed earlier in this chapter, might be all that is needed.

In terms of presentation, no board member or senior manager enjoys wading through voluminous reports in order to find the key business indicators. Similarly, no one enjoys reading or listening to an explanation of operations that focuses on the calculations contained in the statements. For example, the following comments might have accompanied the department report to a senior manager shown in figure 5-2:

> Total department salaries and wages for the month of May amounted to $127,593, or $4,287 better than budget. Much of this positive variance was caused by account 848, X-ray technicians, which was better than budget by $4,217. Offsetting unfavorable variances were. . . .

The comment is redundant, boring, worthless, and generally irritating. It should always be assumed that the senior manager or board member can and will read the background material. The presenter should focus on why a significant variance occurred. For an unfavorable variance, the explanation should show how and by what date the variance will be corrected and the actual results brought in line with the budget. For a favorable variance, the explanation should show how the hospital is going to maintain the favorable variance. The presenter should focus on the effect of significant variances on the services provided by the department or the institution. The senior manager, clinical manager, or department manager should consider whether he or she has been able to improve patient services or obtain better outcomes with fewer resources. If so, the methods should be explained to the board. That would be of real interest to a board member.

A primary theme of this text has been the need for the budget to focus on the institution's goals. Operating reports should show how those goals are being attained and what resources are required to attain them. Attaining the stated goals and improving results are the overall objectives. Progress toward the goals should be reflected in timely, understandable, and informative operating reports.

Appendix

Model Operating Budget

Contents

Note: In addition to the analyses included in this model, a complete budget package would include a summary of the operating plan and sufficient program analyses to show how budget resources would be utilized to attain the operating plan's objectives. The package should also contain a description of how the expenses shown in the accompanying budget analyses would be flexed and reported on the basis of actual activity during the year.

To: The Members of the Board of Directors
General Hospital

From: Steve Jones, President
General Hospital

Subject: Operating Budget—1992

The attached budget package for 1992 has been prepared on the basis of the objectives specifically outlined in the 1992 operating plan. We believe that the proposed resource allocations will accomplish the operating objectives. The measurements determined in the plan will be compared to the results of actual operations during the course of 1992 to ensure that the objectives are attained.

Fiscal year 1992 will be a period of continued stable operations during which we will finalize the plans for an expansion of our inpatient facilities. The new facilities, for which construction is scheduled to begin in 1993, will support our plans for growth in general surgery and cardiac care.

The pressure on our net income resulting from increased discounts to major payers and general inflation will be offset by a 6 percent average rate increase and an increased focus on employee effectiveness. Management's emphasis on the constant improvement of patient service and the monitoring of key quality indicators will ensure that any reduction in personnel or change in responsibility will not adversely affect service quality but will instead result in, or be accompanied by, improved service.

General Hospital—1992 Operating Budget
Income and Expenses

	Reference Page	1991 Budget	1991 Projection	1992 Budget	Increase (Decrease) over 1991 Projection Amount	Percent
Patient service revenue						
Inpatient						
Basic daily hospital charges	171	$11,630,000	$12,281,000	$13,121,000	$ 840,000	6.8
Ancillary services	173	11,423,000	12,216,000	13,548,000	1,332,000	10.9
Total inpatient	171	23,053,000	24,497,000	26,669,000	2,172,000	8.9
Outpatient	171, 173	2,733,000	3,228,000	3,576,000	348,000	10.8
Total patient service revenue		$25,786,000	$27,725,000	$30,245,000	$2,520,000	9.1
Less:						
Medicare/Medicaid allowances	170	$ 2,968,000	$ 3,291,000	$ 3,660,000	$ 369,000	11.2
Blue Cross/other allowances	170	532,000	489,000	545,000	56,000	11.5
Free care and uncollectible accounts less recoveries	174	1,158,000	1,074,000	1,088,000	14,000	1.3
		$ 4,658,000	$ 4,854,000	$ 5,293,000	$ 439,000	9.0
Net patient revenue		$21,128,000	$22,871,000	$24,952,000	$2,081,000	9.1
Other operating revenue	174	481,000	497,000	528,000	31,000	6.2
Net revenue		$21,609,000	$23,368,000	$25,480,000	$2,112,000	9.0
Operating expenses						
Salaries and wages	175	$11,101,000	$12,615,000	$13,910,000	$1,295,000	10.3
Employee benefits	177	1,676,000	1,892,000	1,989,000	97,000	5.1
Supplies and services	178	5,776,000	6,137,000	6,654,000	517,000	8.4
Depreciation	179	1,010,000	1,005,000	1,072,000	67,000	6.7
Insurance	179	668,000	643,000	603,000	(40,000)	(6.2)
Interest	179	262,000	265,000	256,000	(9,000)	(3.4)
Total operating expense		$20,493,000	$22,557,000	$24,484,000	$1,927,000	8.5
Net income		$ 1,116,000	$ 811,000	$ 996,000	$ 185,000	22.8
Percent of net income to total patient service revenue		4.3%	2.9%	3.3%		

General Hospital—1992 Operating Budget
Occupancy Statistics

	Bed Complement	1991 Budget Patient Days	Percent Occupancy	1991 Projection Patient Days	Percent Occupancy	1992 Budget Patient Days	Percent Occupancy
Patient days							
Medical	76	26,131	94.2	26,381	95.1	26,464	95.4
Surgical	101	34,511	93.6	34,248	92.9	34,469	93.5
Intensive care unit	12	2,957	67.5	3,000	68.5	3,009	68.7
Cardiac care unit	12	3,110	71.0	3,035	69.3	3,167	72.3
Pediatrics	15	3,313	60.5	3,028	55.3	3,039	55.5
Obstetrics	22	5,380	67.0	5,525	68.8	5,541	69.0
Total	238	75,402	86.8	75,217	86.6	75,689	87.1
Admissions		9,765		9,897		10,038	
Average length of stay		7.72 days		7.60 days		7.54 days	

General Hospital—1992 Operating Budget
Operating Highlights

Sources of Inpatient Revenue

The patient services revenue is the total gross revenue that would be generated if all patient services were paid in accordance with the published schedule of charges for each service. The estimated distribution, in percent, of the sources of inpatient revenue for the budget year is as follows:

Payment based on schedule of charges:		
Blue Cross and HMO/PPO contracts	14%	
Commercial insurance	35	
Individual patients	7	56%
Payment from federal and state contracts:		
Medicare	28%	
Medicaid and other state-supported agencies	15	43
Payment based on historical cost:		
County general assistance		1
Total		100%

Patient Days

The increase of 472 patient days over the 1991 projections is primarily the result of increased utilization of the operating rooms and the cardiac care unit. There are no new services that would affect the number of patient days.

Medicare/Medicaid and Blue Cross/Other Allowances

Medicare pays for covered services on a per case basis following a schedule of fees for specific diagnosis-related groups (DRGs) of patients. Medicaid pays the hospital on the basis of a per diem rate. The basic rate is adjusted only for psychiatric and rehabilitation patients, who are covered at a lower rate. The negotiated general Medicaid per diem rate for 1992 will be $226.00. The estimated allowances for 1992 are 13.9 percent of total patient services income and 27.5 percent of the estimated inpatient charges for services to Medicare, Medicaid, and other patients covered by federal, state, and local government programs. The allowances for the budget year are higher than the projection primarily due to a change made by Medicare to decrease the level of DRG payment. Blue Cross and most other contract payers pay the hospital on the basis of discounted charges, with certain limitations. The estimated allowance for Blue Cross and others is equal to 12.7 percent of estimated inpatient charges for services to covered contract patients.

Free Care and Uncollectible Accounts Less Recoveries

Free care and uncollectible accounts less recoveries are budgeted at 3.6 percent of total patient services income. This includes 3.2 percent for uncollectible accounts, and the balance is primarily the free care services rendered in the hospital, net of the specific free care endowment income, and other funds restricted for such free care.

Other Operating Revenue

The other operating revenue budgeted for 1992 is $31,000 higher than the 1991 projection. The additional income is primarily from an 8 percent increase in the price of items in the employee cafeteria. The increase was attributable to increased food costs and cafeteria labor costs.

Salaries and Wages

The 1992 budget provides for cost-of-living adjustments of wage scales effective January 1, 1992, and for a merit increase for each employee in the pay period preceding the individual's scheduled annual review date as follows:

	Total	Scale Adjustment	Merit
Clerical	9%	4%	5%
Technical	10	5	5
Nursing	11	4	7
Management	9	4	5
Executive (including salaried physicians)	6	—	6

Employee Benefits

There are no major changes in the present employee benefit plans provided for the 1992 budget. Employee fringe benefits will equal 14.3 percent of total salaries and wages.

Supplies and Services Expense

Supplies and services expense increased by $566,000 (9.22 percent) over the 1991 projection of $6,137,000. The increase is due primarily to price inflation.

Depreciation

A slight increase in depreciation is expected because of new equipment purchases.

Insurance

Insurance expense decreased by $40,000 because of the favorable rates quoted by the professional liability carrier.

General Hospital—1992 Operating Budget

Average per Diem and per Procedure Charges

	Reference Page	1991 Budget	1991 Projection	1992 Budget	Increase (Decrease) over 1991 Projection	
					Amount	Percent
Inpatient per diem						
Basic daily hospital charges		$ 154.24	$ 163.27	$ 173.35	$ 10.08	6.2
Ancillary services		151.50	162.41	179.00	16.59	10.2
Total per diem		$ 305.74	$ 325.68	$ 352.35	$ 26.67	8.2
Patient days		75,402	75,217	75,689	472	0.6
Inpatient charges						
Basic daily hospital charge × patient days	169	$11,630,000	$12,281,000	$13,121,000	$ 840,000	6.8
Ancillary charge × patient days	169	11,423,000	12,216,000	13,548,000	1,332,000	10.9
Total inpatient charges	169	$23,053,000	$24,497,000	$26,669,000	$2,172,000	8.9
Outpatient average charge per procedure		$ 18.52	$ 22.03	$ 23.70	$ 1.67	7.6
Outpatient procedures		147,541	146,552	150,867	4,315	2.9
Outpatient charges	169	$ 2,733,000	$ 3,228,000	$ 3,576,000	$ 348,000	10.8

General Hospital—1992 Operating Budget
Analysis of Increase in Patient Revenue—Price and Volume Changes

Effective January 1, 1992, the average billing will be increased 6 percent at General Hospital. The income variation resulting from this general price increase and volume change is as follows:

	Total	Inpatient	Outpatient
Price increase (effective January 1, 1992)			
Inpatient: Increase in rates averaging $19.51 (6%) per day	$1,470,000	$1,470,000	$ —
Outpatient: Increase in rates for ambulatory care and ancillary services (6%)	194,000	—	194,000
Total price increase	$1,664,000	$1,470,000	$194,000
Volume and intensity			
Inpatient:			
Increase of 472 patient days at an average of $325.68 per day (volume)	$ 157,000	$ 157,000	$ —
Increase in amount of ancillary services used (intensity) has an effect of $7.16 per day for 75,689 days	545,000	545,000	—
Outpatient			
Increased number of visits and increased intensity	154,000	—	154,000
Total volume increase	$ 856,000	$ 702,000	$154,000
Revenue increase	$2,520,000	$2,172,000	$348,000

General Hospital—1992 Operating Budget
Impact of January 1, 1992, Rate Increase

The impact of the average per diem of the January 1, 1992, increase, broken down by area of service, is as follows:

	Impact of January 1, 1992, Increase
Basic daily charge (most common two-bed room rate will be $123.00 as of January 1, 1992)	$ 9.80
Ancillary services	
Operating room	$ 1.42
Central supply	1.02
Intravenous therapy	0.65
Emergency department	0.27
Laboratory	1.88
Blood bank	0.28
Electrocardiogram	0.23
Cardiac catheterization laboratory	0.28
Radiology	0.72
Respiratory therapy	0.46
Pharmacy	1.24
CT scan	0.23
All other	1.03
Total ancillary	$ 9.71
Total	$19.51

General Hospital—1992 Operating Budget
Ancillary Service Revenue

Service	1991 Projection			1992 Budget			Increase	
	Inpatient	Outpatient	Total	Inpatient	Outpatient	Total	Amount	Percent
Operating room	$ 1,775,000	$ 115,000	$ 1,890,000	$ 1,962,000	$ 129,000	$ 2,091,000	$ 201,000	10.6
Recovery room	323,000	6,000	329,000	357,000	7,000	364,000	35,000	10.6
Delivery room	310,000	0	310,000	342,000	0	342,000	32,000	10.3
Central supply	1,282,000	30,000	1,312,000	1,394,000	33,000	1,427,000	115,000	8.8
Intravenous therapy	813,000	20,000	833,000	921,000	21,000	942,000	109,000	13.1
Emergency department	344,000	1,154,000	1,498,000	399,000	1,280,000	1,679,000	181,000	12.1
Anesthesiology	194,000	11,000	205,000	213,000	11,000	224,000	19,000	9.3
Day surgery	2,000	46,000	48,000	5,000	51,000	56,000	8,000	16.7
Laboratory	2,359,000	948,000	3,307,000	2,650,000	999,000	3,649,000	342,000	10.3
Blood bank	346,000	15,000	361,000	371,000	17,000	388,000	27,000	7.5
Electrocardiogram	291,000	32,000	323,000	322,000	35,000	357,000	34,000	10.5
Cardiac catheterization	355,000	47,000	402,000	426,000	52,000	478,000	76,000	18.9
Radiology	896,000	595,000	1,491,000	969,000	652,000	1,621,000	130,000	8.7
Ultrasound	34,000	11,000	45,000	35,000	21,000	56,000	11,000	24.4
Electroencephalogram	57,000	11,000	68,000	63,000	11,000	74,000	6,000	8.8
Respiratory therapy	573,000	23,000	596,000	634,000	24,000	658,000	62,000	10.4
Physical therapy	274,000	67,000	341,000	304,000	74,000	378,000	37,000	10.9
Pharmacy	1,551,000	58,000	1,609,000	1,714,000	64,000	1,778,000	169,000	10.5
Nuclear medicine	146,000	23,000	169,000	161,000	26,000	187,000	18,000	10.7
CT scan	291,000	16,000	307,000	306,000	69,000	375,000	68,000	22.1
	$12,216,000	$ 3,228,000	$15,444,000	$13,548,000	$3,576,000	$17,124,000	$1,680,000	10.9

—— Reference page 169 ——   —— Reference page 169 ——

General Hospital—1992 Operating Budget
Free Care and Uncollectible Accounts Less Recoveries

	1991 Budget	1991 Projection	1992 Budget
Free care	$ 115,000	$ 111,000	$ 120,000
Uncollectible accounts	1,155,000	1,061,000	1,092,000
Recoveries of uncollectible accounts	(112,000)	(98,000)	(124,000)
Net write-offs (reference page 169)	$ 1,158,000	$ 1,074,000	$ 1,088,000
Total patient service revenue	$25,786,000	$27,725,000	$30,245,000
Net write-offs to revenue (%)	4.5%	3.9%	3.6%

Note: In 1992 General Hospital is required under Hill–Burton charity regulations to provide free care in the amount of $43,000 (10 percent of the grant received in 1965). By the end of fiscal year 1992, General Hospital will have met the total obligation required by the regulation.

General Hospital—1992 Operating Budget
Other Operating Revenue

	1991 Budget	1991 Projection	1992 Budget	Increase (Decrease)	
				Price	Volume
Investment income	$ 3,000	$ 5,000	$ 3,000		$(2,000)
Cafeteria	128,000	135,000	146,000	$11,000	—
Coffee shop	62,000	58,000	63,000	5,000	—
Gift shop	132,000	135,000	150,000	14,000	1,000
Telephone	3,000	3,000	3,000	—	—
Record reprints	10,000	9,000	11,000	—	2,000
Data-processing services	28,000	33,000	32,000	—	(1,000)
Parking	40,000	43,000	44,000	—	1,000
Professional building rental	64,000	64,000	71,000	6,000	1,000
Miscellaneous	11,000	12,000	5,000	—	(7,000)
	$481,000	$497,000	$528,000	$36,000	$(5,000)

————— Reference page 169 —————

General Hospital—1992 Operating Budget
Analysis of Salaries and Wages

The 1992 budget for salaries and wages includes the following:

Salaries and Wages	Average Salary	Number of Full-Time Equivalent Employees	Dollar Amount
Nurses (R.N., L.P.N., and others)	$19,800	226	$ 4,475,000
Hourly employees	15,915	198	3,151,000
Management and salaried physicians	36,247	14	508,000
Clerical, technical, and administrative	18,980	295	5,599,000
Temporary employees	—	—	73,000
Summer salaries	—	—	19,000
Overtime	—	—	339,000
Vacancy allowance	—	—	(254,000)
Total	$18,976	733	$13,910,000

Reference
page 169

General Hospital—1992 Operating Budget
Analysis of Salaries and Wages

The increase from 1991 projected salary and wage expense is as follows:

	Number of Full-Time Equivalent Employees	Increase (Decrease)		Dollar Amount
		Percent	Amount	
1991 projection	724			$12,615,000
Cost-of-living adjustment on January 1, 1992		4.0	$ 505,000	505,000
Merit-increase program		5.7	715,000	715,000
Annualized effect of new positions added during 1991. All were included in 1991 budget. (Reference page 176)	9	0.9	84,000	84,000
Annualized effect of positions deleted during 1991	(5)	(0.7)	(89,000)	(89,000)
Effect of new positions authorized in 1992 budget (Reference page 176)	5	0.9	80,000	80,000
1992 budget	733	10.3	$1,295,000	$13,910,000

Reference
page 169

General Hospital—1992 Operating Budget
Analysis of Salaries and Wages

Positions added in 1991 anticipated to be filled during the entire year (1992) have the impact of an increase in that the budget for a full-year salary is compared to the current or expected salaries for less than a full year. The following positions account for the increase:

Department	Full-Time Equivalent	Job Description	Amount of Increase
Nursing administration	1.0	Supervisor/assistant	$12,000
Medical-surgical nursing	1.7	R.N./L.P.N.	23,000
Operating room	1.0	R.N.	6,000
Radiology	2.0	X-ray technician	18,000
CT scan	1.0	X-ray technician	13,000
Dietary	2.0	Dietitian	12,000
			$84,000

Reference page 175

The following new positions have been requested for 1992:

Department	Requested as a result of:				Amount of Increase
	New Services		Additional Work Load		
	Full-Time Equivalent	Description	Full-Time Equivalent	Description	
Medical-surgical nursing		—	1.5	Nurses	$19,000
Cardiac care unit		—	1.0	Nurse	14,000
Recovery room		On-call program	—		13,000
Laboratory	1.5	Medical technicians	1.0	Supervisor	34,000
					$80,000

Reference page 175

The following positions were eliminated in 1991 and will have the impact of decreased salary and wage expense in 1992:

Department	Full-time Equivalent	Job Description	Amount of Decrease
Administration	2	Assistant administrator	$45,000
Administration	1	Secretary	11,000
Administration	1	Administrative assistant	16,000
Security	1	Security officer	17,000
			$89,000

General Hospital—1992 Operating Budget
Analysis of Employee Benefits (000 Omitted)

Employee fringe benefits include the following

Fringe Benefits	1991 Budget		1991 Projection		1992 Budget	
	Amount (000 Omitted)	Percent of Salaries	Amount	Percent of Salaries	Amount	Percent of Salaries
Social Security taxes	$ 577	5.2	$ 675	5.4	$ 751[a]	5.4
Pension plans	377	3.4	410	3.3	362[b]	2.6
Unemployment compensation	111	1.0	126	1.0	125[c]	0.9
Workers' compensation	56	0.5	63	0.5	70[d]	0.5
Life and disability	56	0.5	63	0.4	70[e]	0.5
Blue Cross/Blue Shield	455	4.1	517	4.1	570[f]	4.1
Employee medical services	44	0.4	38	0.3	41	0.3
	$1,676	15.1	$1,892	15.0	$1,989	14.3
	Reference page 169		Reference page 169		Reference page 169	

[a] An increase in salary expense and an increase in the taxable wage base to $48,000 as of January 1, 1992. The rate will remain at 7.65 percent.

[b] Based on current actuarial figures. The 1991 projection includes some additional expenses required to update the plan to meet new ERISA requirements.

[c] Based on the most recent 12 months (July 1, 1990, to June 30, 1991) experience of $72,000, plus a 30 percent projected increase for budget year 1992.

[d] The bulk of this expense is small claims administered by ABC, Inc. In the same 12 months ending June 30, 1991, they paid out $42,000. This year's budget is based on a 25 percent increase. The remaining increase is attributable to increased service fees and the increased costs of the aggregate loss policies.

[e] The basic amount of free life insurance was increased from $8,000 to $10,000 for each full-time employee, and the rate for salary continuance insurance was increased 1.5 cents per $100 of covered monthly salaries.

[f] The 1992 Blue Cross budget is based on actual 1990 calendar year claims plus 27.7 percent, which reflects the actual increase in claim experience over the past two years.

General Hospital—1992 Operating Budget
Supplies and Services Expense

	Notes	1991 Budget	1991 Projection	1992 Budget	Increase (Decrease) from 1991 Projection	Increase (Decrease) because of Price	Increase (Decrease) because of Volume
Medical supplies (1)	1	$ 920,000	$1,101,000	$1,179,000	$517,000	$115,000	$(37,000)
Drugs, films, and solutions (2)	2	724,000	748,000	820,000	72,000	66,000	6,000
Commissions and fees	3	718,000	752,000	812,000	60,000	22,000	38,000
Utilities	4	467,000	475,000	539,000	64,000	64,000	–
Food	5	457,000	478,000	536,000	58,000	54,000	4,000
General administrative	6	438,000	465,000	527,000	62,000	57,000	5,000
Rentals	7	428,000	434,000	463,000	29,000	29,000	–
Professional services	8	370,000	393,000	430,000	37,000	35,000	2,000
Laundry and linen	9	233,000	248,000	260,000	12,000	5,000	7,000
Service contracts	10	227,000	231,000	255,000	24,000	17,000	7,000
Building and equipment	11	187,000	188,000	176,000	(12,000)	–	(12,000)
Telephone	12	139,000	148,000	158,000	10,000	10,000	–
Other	13	468,000	476,000	499,000	23,000	23,000	–
Total		$5,776,000	$6,137,000	$6,654,000	$517,000	$497,000	$ 20,000

Reference page 169

Notes to Supplies and Services Expense:

1. *Medical supplies.* There has been a continuing significant increase in the usage and the cost of medical supplies over the past several years. The large increase of 1991 projection over the budget is because of volume. Management bought larger quantities during the current year in anticipation of even greater cost escalation in 1991. Included in the 1992 budget is an average price increase for medical supplies of 10.5 percent. The new services column shown below refers to the pacemaker implant program ($7,000), projected to begin in the second half of the year, and the cardiovascular health maintenance program ($5,000).

		Increase (Decrease) over 1991 Projection	
		Volume	
Account	Price	New Services	Current Services
Disposable linen	$ 9,000	–	$ 5,000
Medical and surgical instruments	4,000	–	–
Radioactive material	3,000	–	–
Supplies charged to patients	–	7,000	–
Laboratory supplies	2,000	–	–
Medical and surgical supplies	97,000	5,000	(54,000)
	$115,000	$12,000	$(49,000)

2. *Drugs, films, and solutions.* This note and others (through 13) would contain a detailed analysis of the variance, as shown in note 1.

General Hospital—1992 Operating Budget
Depreciation

	1991 Budget	1991 Projection	1992 Budget	Increase (Decrease) from 1991 Projection	
				Amount	Percent
Buildings	$ 537,000[a]	$ 532,000	$ 542,000	$10,000	1.9
Equipment	478,000[b]	473,000	530,000	57,000	12.1
	$1,015,000	$1,005,000	$1,072,000	$67,000	6.7

———————————— Reference on page 169 ————————————

Note: Depreciation for both buildings and equipment was calculated using an accelerated method for acquisitions before January 1, 1968, and subsequent additions on a straight-line basis. Equipment is depreciated over a 10-year period, which represents a composite life for all equipment. Buildings, in general, are depreciated over a 40-year period, except for some older facilities that are being written off over a much shorter life. Generally, one-half year's depreciation is taken in the year of addition.

[a] Committed to finance construction of new facilities and pay principal payments on long-term debt.
[b] Committed for equipment replacement, additions, and renovations.

General Hospital—1992 Operating Budget
Insurance

	1991 Budget	1991 Projection	1992 Budget	Increase (Decrease) from 1991 Projection	
				Amount	Percentage
Fire and extended coverage	$ 26,000	$ 21,000	$ 24,000	$ 3,000	14.3
Professional and public liability	642,000	622,000	$579,000	(43,000)	(6.9)
Total	$668,000	$643,000	$603,000	$(40,000)	(6.2)

———————————— Reference page 169 ————————————

General Hospital—1992 Operating Budget
Interest

	Principal Balance 12/31/91	Principal Payments 1992	Interest Expense
Bonds, series 1986, 6 to 6.75%, maturing in increasing annual amounts through 2006	$4,452,000	$167,000	$276,000
Interest recovery on deposits to "principal and interest funds"			(31,000)
Deferred bond issue expenses			7,000
Capitalized lease agreements maturing in increasing monthly amounts until 2002	90,000	48,000	4,000
Total	$4,542,000	$215,000	$256,000

Reference page 169

General Hospital—1992 Operating Budget
Balance Sheet—Projected 1991, Budget 1992

Assets	Projected 1991	Budget 1992
Current assets		
Cash investments	$ 300,000	$ 500,000
Patient services receivables, net of allowances of $360,000 in 1991 and $407,000 in 1992	3,240,000	3,661,000
Due from Medicare and Medicaid	177,000	177,000
Other accounts receivable	130,000	100,000
Other current assets	414,000	490,000
Total current assets	$ 4,261,000	$ 4,928,000
Property and equipment		
Land and buildings	$14,594,000	$14,620,000
Movable equipment	4,156,000	5,006,000
Construction in process	106,000	246,000
	$18,856,000	$19,872,000
Less: accumulated depreciation	(5,250,000)	(6,322,000)
Total property and equipment	$13,606,000	$13,550,000
Funds designated for future expansion	$ 1,668,000	$ 2,258,000
Endowment and other restricted investments	$1,340,000	$ 1,360,000
Total assets	$20,875,000	$22,096,000

Liabilities and Fund Balances	Projected 1991	Budget 1992
Current liabilities		
Accounts payable	$ 300,000	$ 500,000
Salaries, wages, and other accruals	460,000	680,000
Portion of long-term debt due within one year	215,000	255,000
Total current liabilities	$ 975,000	$ 1,435,000
Long-term debt, less current portion	$ 2,900,000	$ 2,645,000
Fund balances		
Unrestricted funds	$15,660,000	$16,656,000
Endowment and other restricted funds	1,340,000	1,360,000
Total fund balances	$17,000,000	$18,016,000
Total liabilities and fund balances	$20,875,000	$22,096,000

General Hospital—1992 Operating Budget
Changes in Financial Position—Budget 1992

Cash and investments, beginning of 1992		$ 300,000
Funds provided from:		
Net income	$ 996,000	
Depreciation	1,072,000	
Total cash from operations		2,068,000
Endowment donation		20,000
Increase in accounts payable		200,000
Increase in salaries, wages, and other accruals		220,000
Decrease in other accounts receivables		30,000
Total funds available		$2,838,000
Funds applied to:		
Increase in accounts receivable		$ 421,000
Increase in other assets		76,000
Increase in property and equipment		1,016,000
Increase in funds designated for future expansion		590,000
Payment on long-term debt		215,000
Increase in endowment and other restricted investments		20,000
Total funds applied		2,338,000
Cash and investments, end of 1992		$ 500,000

General Hospital—1992 Operating Budget
Capital Budget 1992

Cost Center Item Description[a] (Quantity)	Month of Purchase	Total Cost	Estimated Payment ($)			
			First Quarter	Second Quarter	Third Quarter	Fourth Quarter
Medicine—2 East						
Wheelchairs (2)	Feb.		$ 950	$ —	$ —	$ —
Defibrillator	May	11,900	—	11,900	—	—
Medicine—2 West						
In-bed scale	Jan.	3,500	3,500	—	—	
Refrigerator	Nov.	400	—	—	—	400
Surgery—3 West						
Ice machine	Oct.	2,500	—	—	—	2,500
Secretary chairs (2)	Sept.	900	—	—	900	—
Laboratory						
Bloodcell separator	Aug.	5,900	—	—	5,900	—
Microscope	June	2,700	—	2,700	—	—
Laminar flow hood	April	5,000	—	5,000	—	—
Dietary						
Deep fryer	March	400	400	—	—	—
Microwaves (4)	April/May	3,200	—	3,200	—	—
	Sept./Nov.	3,200	—	—	1,600	1,600
Four-drawer file	July	250	—	—	250	—
Finance						
Computers (2)	Feb./May	4,800	2,400	2,400	—	—
Computer disk	Aug.	13,000	—	—	13,000	—
Calculators (2)	Feb./May	1,200	600	600	—	—
Housekeeping						
.	.	.	.	.	.	.
.	.	.	.	.	.	.
.	.	.	.	.	.	.
Construction and Hospital Maintenance						
Recarpet cafeteria	Dec.	7,000	—	—	—	7,000
Install sprinkler system in lab	Jan.	16,000	16,000	—	—	
Totals		$1,016,000	$250,000	$258,000	$256,000	$252,000

[a]This is a partial list for format presentation only.

General Hospital—1992 Operating Budget
Capital Budget 1993–1994

Cost Center	Item Description (Quantity)[a]	1993	1994
Intensive care unit	Television monitoring of rooms 143 and 144; mass spectrometry	$ 3,000	$ 4,500
Cardiac care unit	Television monitoring of rooms 145 and 146; mass spectrometry	3,000	4,500
Nursery	pH monitors	11,000	
Intravenous therapy	Remodel area	7,000	
	Clean air hood	3,000	
Anesthesia	Anesthesia machines (2)	16,000	
	Anesthesia machines (2)		17,000
Radiology	Fluoroscopy unit	200,000	
	Multidirectional tomography unit	260,000	
	Trauma chest unit		150,000
Physical therapy	Diathermy	3,000	
	Treadmill bike	5,800	
Ultrasound	Small-parts real-time unit	90,000	
Maintenance	Window screens for patient rooms	4,700	
	Window screens for patient rooms		4,700
Linen room	Washing machine	8,000	
Dietary	Microwaves (4)	6,800	
	Microwaves (2)		3,800
Coffee shop	Tables, chairs, drapery, and carpet		7,000
Purchasing	Electrical power forklift truck	3,500	
	Televisions (100)	35,500	
	Televisions (100)		35,500
		$860,300	$627,000

[a]This is a partial list for format presentation only.

Bibliography

Abendshien, J. *A Guide to the Board's Role in Strategic Business Planning.* Chicago: American Hospital Publishing, 1988.

Annis, R. Budgeting: getting to the bottom line. *Health Progress* 69(11):74, 76, Dec. 1988.

Baird, P. J., and Kazamek, T. J. Moving to micro-based cost accounting. *Computers in Healthcare* 9(3):29–31, Mar. 1988.

Baptist, A. J., Saylor, J., and Zerwekh, J. Developing a solid base for a cost accounting system. *Healthcare Financial Management* 41(1):42–48, Jan. 1987.

Berg, D. A search for soul: strategic planning will chart the way. *Health Progress* 70(3):38–41, Apr. 1989.

Birch, S., and Donaldson, C. Cost-benefit analysis: dealing with problems of indivisible projects and fixed budgets. *Health Policy* 7(1):61–72, Feb. 1987.

Brady, F. J. Labor of love: a model for planning human resource needs. *Health Progress* 70(6):78–81, July–Aug. 1989.

Broering, N. C. *Strategic Planning: An Integrated Academic Information Management System (IAIMS) at Georgetown University Medical Center.* Washington, DC: Georgetown University Medical Center, 1986.

Camillus, J. C. *The Practice of Strategic Planning.* New York City: National League for Nursing, 1980.

Cleverley, W. O. Strategic financial planning: a balance sheet perspective. *Hospital and Health Services Administration* 32(1):1–20, Feb. 1987.

Cleverley, W. O. Ten financial management principles for survival. *Health Progress* 69(2):36–41, 104, Mar. 1988.

This bibliography was compiled from the Health Planning and Administration Data Base, which was cooperatively produced by the National Library of Medicine and the American Hospital Association Resource Center.

Cleverley, W. O. How boards can use comparative data in strategic planning. *Health-care Executive* 4(3):32–33, May–June 1989.

Counte, M. A., and Glandon, G. L. Managerial innovation in the hospital: an analysis of the diffusion of hospital cost-accounting systems. *Hospital and Health Services Administration* 33(3):371–84, Fall 1988.

Coyne, J. S. Corporate cash management in health care: can we do better? *Healthcare Financial Management* 41(9):76–79, Sept. 1987.

Cronin, F. J., and Goodspeed, S. W. Beyond strategic planning: vision, mission, strategy are three steps to success. *Healthcare Executive* 3(3):28–31, May–June 1988.

Deets, M. K. Bridging the gap between strategic planning and the budget. *Trustee* 40(9):10–12, Sept. 1987.

Department of Hospital Planning and Society for Hospital Planning of the American Hospital Association. *Compendium of Resources for Strategic Planning in Hospitals*. Chicago: American Hospital Association, 1981.

Dieter, B. B. Flexible budgeting in healthcare. *Computers in Healthcare* 8(3):71–72, Mar. 1987.

Dillon, R. D. *Zero-Base Budgeting for Health Care Institutions*. Germantown, MD: Aspen Systems Corporation, 1979.

Doyle, O. Healthcare executives should prepare for implementation of cost accounting. *Modern Healthcare* 18(36): 60, Sept. 2, 1988.

Eastaugh, S. R. Has PPS affected the sophistication of cost accounting? *Healthcare Financial Management* 41(11):50–53, Nov. 1987.

Evashwick, C. J., and Evashwick, W. T. The fine art of strategic planning. *Provider* 14(4):4–6, Apr. 1988.

Fagin, C. M. Strategic planning: outline of plan. *Journal of Professional Nursing* 3(2):79, 124, Mar.–Apr. 1987.

Finkler, S. A., Williams, S. V., and Eisenberg, J. M. *Current Issues in Hospital Cost Accounting*. Philadelphia: National Health Care Management Center, University of Pennsylvania, 1981.

Flexner, W. A., Berkowitz, E. N., and Brown, M. *Strategic Planning in Health Care Management*. Rockville, MD: Aspen Systems Corporation, 1981.

Folger, J. C. Integration of strategic, financial plans vital to success. *Healthcare Financial Management* 43(1):23, 26–28, 30–32, Jan. 1989.

Fournet, B. A. *Strategic Business Planning in Health Services Management*. Rockville, MD: Aspen Systems Corporation, 1982.

Gallina, J. N. Tips and techniques: application of strategic planning techniques for short-term results. *Current Concepts in Hospital Pharmacy Management* 11(1):14–16, Spring 1989.

Gay, E. G., Kronenfeld, J. J., Baker, S. L., and Amidon, R.L. An appraisal of organizational response to fiscally constraining regulation: the case of hospitals and DRGs. *Journal of Health and Social Behavior* 30(1):41–55, Mar. 1989.

Gragg, J. H., and Johnson, J. L. Cost accounting: alive and well for the 1990s. *U.S. Healthcare* 6(4):36, 38, 40, Apr. 1989.

Graham, N. G. Self-governing hospitals: a hospital manager's assessment. *British Journal of Hospital Medicine* 42(3):234–36, Sept. 1989.

Greaf, W. D. Strategic planning: is it still useful? *DRG Monitor* 6(10):1–8, June 1989.

Groth, C. D. Business growth through strategic planning. *Group Practice Journal* 36(2):42–45, Mar.–Apr. 1987.

Harris, J., and Pitts, K. Capital management helps hospitals face hard times. *Healthcare Financial Management* 43(3):21–22, 26, 28, Mar. 1989.

Hatcher, M. E., and Connelly, C. A case mix simulation decision support system model for negotiating hospital rates. *Journal of Medical Systems* 12(6):341–63, Dec. 1988.

Hawkins, B., Needham, K., and Briggs, I. Budget analysis needed expert eye. *Health Service Journal* 99(5153): suppl. 8, 10, June 1, 1989.

Hemeon, F. E., 3rd. Productivity, cost accounting, and information systems. *Topics in Health Care Financing* 15(3):55–67, Spring 1989.

Herkimer, A. G., Jr. *Understanding Health Care Budgeting.* Rockville, MD: Aspen Systems Corporation, 1988.

Hogan, J. M., ed. *Strategic Planning and Marketing.* Gaithersburg, MD: Aspen Systems Corporation, 1986.

Hospital Research and Educational Trust of the American Hospital Association and Society for Healthcare Planning and Marketing. *Environmental Assessment Workbook: Identifying the Hospital's Local Issues.* Chicago: American Hospital Publishing, 1989.

Javor, A., Kovacs, J., and Suli, J. A reform concept for performance assessment and cost accounting in health care. *Sante Publique (Bucur)* 32(2):129–38, Apr.–June 1989.

Jennings, M. C. What is financially driven strategic planning? *Topics in Health Care Financing* 15(1):1–8, Fall 1988.

Johnson, R. R., and McGinty, D. G. Product line management requires change in financial reports. *Healthcare Financial Management* 43(8):34, 36, 38, Aug. 1989.

Jones, R. A. Taking the "guesstimates" out of FTE budgeting: full-time equivalency. *Nursing Management* 20(2):65–66, 68, 72–73, Feb. 1989.

Jones, W. J. Reality-based strategies for real times. *Health Care Strategic Management* 7(6):16–18, June 1989.

Kamath, R. R., and Elmer, J. Capital investment decisions in hospitals: survey results. *Health Care Management Review* 14(2):45–56, Spring 1989.

Kaskiw, E. A., Hanlon, P., and Wulf, P. Cost accounting in health care: fad or fundamental? *Hospital and Health Services Administration* 32(4):457–74, Nov. 1987.

Katz, P. M., and Lohman, P. Niche systems help hospitals manage useful data. *Healthcare Financial Management* 42(11):66–68, Nov. 1988.

Kazamek, T. J. Moving to product line budgeting. *Computers in Healthcare* 9(11):30–32, 34, Nov. 1988.

Kerschner, M. I., and Loper, E. L. Enhancing cost accounting efforts by improving existing information sources. *Topics in Health Care Financing* 13(4):10–19, Summer 1987.

Kerschner, M. I., and Rooney, J. M. Utilizing cost accounting information for budgeting. *Topics in Health Care Financing* 13(4):56–66, Summer 1987.

Kirk, R. *Nurse Staffing and Budgeting: Practical Management Tools.* Rockville, MD: Aspen Systems Corporation, 1986.

Kirk, R. *Healthcare Staffing and Budgeting: Practical Management Tools.* Rockville, MD: Aspen Systems Corporation, 1988.

Kis, G. M., and Bodenger, G. Cost management information improves financial performance. *Healthcare Financial Management* 43(5):36, 38, 40–42, May 1989.

Knapp, M. T., DeAngelis, P. L., Jr. Strategic planning vital to eldercare diversification. *Healthcare Financial Management* 43(9):22–26, 28, Sept. 1989.

Krueger, D. J., and Davidson, T. A. Alternative approaches to cost accounting. *Topics in Health Care Financing* 13(4):1–9, Summer 1987.

Kukla, S. F. *Cost Accounting and Financial Analysis for the Hospital Administrator.* Chicago: American Hospital Publishing, 1986.

Ladd, R. D., and Feverstein, T. M. The future of cost accounting systems in healthcare. *Healthcare Computing and Communications* 4(7):62–64, July 1987.

Lampiris, L. Cost accounting and decision support systems: at odds or as a team? *Healthcare Computing and Communications* 5(6):8, 11, June 1988.

Larkin, H. Integrating strategic and financial planning in the hospital. *Trustee* 42(9):14, Sept. 1989.

Larsen, E. R. Systems support cost accounting and quality of care. *Healthcare Financial Management* 42(2):86, 88, Feb. 1988.

Lohrmann, G.M. Flexible budget system a practical approach to cost management. *Healthcare Financial Management* 43(1):38, 40, 44–47, Jan. 1989.

Loria, L. Strategic planning techniques. *Texas Hospitals* 43(8):23–24, Jan. 1988.

Lutz, S. This 10-step process makes rural strategic planning less forbidding. *Modern Healthcare* 19(29):46–47, July 1989.

Margrif, F. D. Getting to the bottom line: hospitals' survival may hinge on the contribution margin. *Health Progress* 70(6):42–45, July–Aug. 1989.

McCutcheon, D. J. Impact analysis reduces the guesswork in budgeting. *Dimensions in Health Services* 65(8):24–25, Nov. 1988.

McGrail, G. R. Budgets: an underused resource. *Journal of Nursing Administration* 18(11):25–31, Nov. 1988.

Mendenhall, S. Integrating clinical, financial information: improving patient management. *Healthcare Financial Management* 42(6):54, 56, 58–60, June 1988.

Mendenhall, S., Shepherd, R., and Kobrinski, E. Cost accounting in healthcare organizations: who needs it? *Healthcare Financial Management* 41(1):34–40, Jan. 1987.

Neff, M. L. General concepts of incremental and zero-based budgeting. *ANNA Journal* 15(6):342–44, Dec. 1988.

O'Connor, N. Integrating patient classification with cost accounting. *Nursing Management* 19(10):27–29, Oct. 1988.

Patterson, P. P. Cost accounting in hospitals and clinical laboratories: Part III. Implementing a real-world system. *Clinical Laboratory Management Review* 3(3):151–56, May–June 1989.

Patterson, P. P. Cost accounting in hospitals and clinical laboratories: Part II. Technical tools for cost accounting. *Clinical Laboratory Management Review* 3(1):26–33, Jan.–Feb. 1989.

Pendola, C. J. *Hospital Budgeting: A Case Study Approach.* Hicksville, NY: Exposition Press, 1976.

Peters, J. A. *A Strategic Planning Process for Hospitals.* Chicago: American Hospital Publishing, 1985.

Picha, P. K. The nursing link to cost accounting. *Nursing Management* 19(5):81, 84, May 1988.

Pivnicny, V. C. Integrating financial and strategic planning. *Health Care Strategic Management* 7(9):14–16, Sept. 1989.

Rathwell, T. *Strategic Planning in the Health Sector.* London: Croom Helm, 1987.

Reeves, R. N., ed. *Strategic Planning for Hospitals.* Chicago: Foundation of the American College of Hospital Administrators, 1983.

Reynolds, M. Management budgeting. *Nursing (London)* 3(23):881–82, Nov. 1987.

Rhoads, J. L. *Basic Accounting and Budgeting for Long-Term Care Facilities.* Boston: CBI, 1981.

Robinson, M. L. Cost accounting slow to influence hospital pricing. *Hospitals* 62(23):18, 20, Dec. 5, 1988.

Rosenbaum, H. L., Willert, T. M., Kelly, E. A., Grey, J. F., and McDonald, B. R. Costing out nursing services based on acuity. *Journal of Nursing Administration* 18(7–8):10–15, July–Aug. 1988.

Sabin, P. Hospital cost accounting and the new imperative. *Hospital Topics* 65(5):33–37, Sept.–Oct. 1987.

Sabin, P. Hospital cost accounting and the new imperative. *Health Progress* 68(4):52–57, May 1987.

Salmen, R. Developing price, charge, and cost rationales. *Hospital Materiel Management Quarterly* 9(1):20–27, Aug. 1987.

Samuels, D. Management: balancing the budget. *Nursing Times* 85(17):34–35, Apr.26–May2, 1989.

Schimmel, V. E., Alley, C., and Heath, A. M. Measuring costs: product line accounting versus ratio of cost to charges. *Topics in Health Care Financing* 13(4):76–86, Summer 1987.

Schlosser, J. R. Strategies for achieving sustained competitive advantage. *Health Care Strategic Management* 5(6):9–13, June 1987.

Schmitz, V., Masters, G. M., and Dilts, W. Better forecasting ensures profitability, quality of care. *Healthcare Financial Management* 43(1):60, 62, 64–66, Jan. 1989.

Schroeder, D. H. Toward a departmental bottom-line perspective. *Health Care Management Review* 14(1):25–40, Winter 1989.

Smith, C. T. Strategic planning and entrepreneurism in academic health centers. *Hospital and Health Service Administration* 33(2):143–52, Summer 1988.

Solovy, A. Hospitals must budget by DRGs, payers. *Hospitals* 63(11):34–37, 39, June 5, 1989.

Stacey, S., and Leggat, S. Strategic planning: a practical guide. *Health Management Forum* 8(2):41–51, Summer 1987.

Stearns, F. E., Jr., and Pinigis, M. Using quality measures with cost accounting for progressive hospital management. *Healthcare Computing and Communications* 5(3):28–29, 32, Mar. 1988.

Stiefel, R. H. Use of a spreadsheet to develop and track budget performance. *Journal of Clinical Engineering* 12(2):133–37, Mar.–Apr. 1987.

Suver, J. D., and Cooper, J. C. Principles and methods of managerial cost-accounting systems. *American Journal of Hospital Pharmacy* 45(1):146–52, Jan. 1988.

Traska, M. R. Managing to the budget means reorienting daily operations. *Hospitals* 62(7):32, Apr. 5, 1988.

Travis, J. F. Bottom-up cost accounting system: a superior method for controlling healthcare costs. *Modern Healthcare* 17(26):50, Dec. 18, 1987.

Trost, A. Steps to sound strategic planning. *Volunteer Leader* 30(3):6–7, Fall 1989.

Tselepis, J. N. Refined cost accounting produces better information. *Healthcare Financial Management* 43(5):26–28, 30, 34, May 1989.

Weiner, S. L., Maxwell, J. H., Sapolsky, H. M., Dunn, D. L., and Hsiao, W. C. Economic incentives and organizational realities: managing hospitals under DRGs. *Milbank Quarterly* 65(4):463–87, 1987.

Wright, K. Financial budgeting: monitoring specialties without specialty costing. *Health Service Journal* 97(5049):532–33, May 7, 1987.

Zipin, M. D. Developing a strategic marketing plan. Health Care Strategic Management 7(6):13–15, June 1989.

Glossary

Accounting cost. The results of transactions as recorded and reported following generally accepted guidelines, conventions, and doctrines. An example of historical accounting cost is the use of depreciation as the systematic and rational allocation of an asset's historical cost over its expected useful life.

Accrual-basis accounting. System for recording transactions. Revenue is recorded in the accounting period in which it is earned, and expenses are recorded in the accounting period in which they are used or consumed in producing revenue. By contrast, the cash basis for recording transactions recognizes revenue only when cash is received and expenses only when cash is disbursed. Under the accrual system, the cost of an asset is expensed (offset against revenue) systematically over its useful life. Under the cash basis, the asset is expensed when it is paid for.

Allowances. Difference between gross revenue from services rendered and amounts received (or to be received) from patients or third-party payers. Allowances most often arise from contractual arrangements with certain large third-party payers. These arrangements provide for a discount for services provided to patients covered by the payer.

Ancillary services. Services provided to patients by the various specialty departments of the hospital, such as radiology, laboratory, pharmacy, or physical therapy, as distinguished from daily nursing care.

Appropriation budget. Type of budget commonly associated with government agencies and characterized by an authorized spending level for a specific period. Revenue estimates are prepared after expenditures are determined. Often the authorized spending level becomes a maximum, and there is a tendency to spend the full amount authorized.

Break-even level. Volume of revenue at which revenue and expenses are exactly equal, that is, the level of activity at which there is neither a gain nor a loss from operations.

Budget. Document that identifies the expected resources and expenditures for a given future period and reflects the nature and source of these resources and expenditures.

Budget calendar. Document showing dates when various steps in the budget process are begun and completed.

Capital asset. Asset costing more than a specific minimum amount and having a life of more than one year. Also, a capital asset is not bought and sold in the ordinary course of hospital operations. A supply item or other inventory-type asset is not a capital asset.

Capital budget. Plan that identifies anticipated purchases of capital assets and the expected source of funds required to make the purchases.

Cash budget. Document that summarizes cash receipts and cash disbursements for regular intervals, usually one month, during the budget year and projects the cash balances at the end of each interval.

Cash flow. Cash receipts less cash disbursements. Cash flow is calculated from an accrual-basis income statement as the excess of revenue over expenses plus depreciation and amortization.

Charity allowances. Difference between full charges and amounts received from, or on behalf of, patients unable to pay.

Contractual adjustments or allowances. Difference between charges and amounts received from third-party payers having special contractual agreements (*see* **Allowances**).

Controllable expense. Expense whose amount is controllable in the short run by someone in the organization, usually a department manager. These expenses are usually variable and form the basis for responsibility accounting.

Cost center. Organizational unit for which revenue and expenses are accumulated separately in the accounts.

Cost-finding analysis. Process of allocating the costs of the non–revenue-producing departments to one another and to the revenue-producing departments on the basis of statistical data that measure the amount of service rendered by each department to the other departments (*see* **Step-down distribution**).

Courtesy allowances. Difference between charges and amounts received from physicians, clergy, employees, and employees' dependents. Also known as policy discounts.

Debt service coverage. Capital-structure ratio that helps a hospital measure its ability to add or increase debt financing and assess its long-term solvency or liquidity. Debt service coverage is defined as cash flow and interest expense divided by principal payment and interest.

Department. Cost center or group of cost centers with one person given responsibility for operations. Also referred to as a responsibility center. This organizational unit is used mostly for internal reporting purposes.

Depreciation expense. Portion of the original cost of a tangible capital asset allocated to a specific accounting period. Because the capital asset has an expected useful life of more than one year, the allocation matches the expense of generating revenue for a specific period to the revenue generated. The alternative is to expense the full amount of an asset's cost in the period the asset was purchased.

Economic cost. An expansion of the accounting cost convention to include such items as depreciation based on replacement cost, rather than historical cost, in the reported expenses. The stated purpose of such a modification is to show the current requirements of an ongoing business in the expense categories rather than include them in the unreported calculation of a minimal net income.

Equivalent occupied beds. A measure in which the hospital inpatient census has been adjusted to reflect an equivalent statistic for outpatient services. The calculation to adjust the average census is:

$$\text{Equivalent occupied beds} = \left(\frac{\text{inpatient revenue} + \text{outpatient revenue}}{\text{inpatient revenue}}\right) \times \text{average census}$$

In the calculation the revenues and average census reflect the activity for the same period.

Expense budget. Document that identifies planned expenditures based on forecasted units of service in the statistical budget. Because of the relative importance of personnel expenditures, the process of translating service statistics into expenses usually is divided into two separate components: the personnel budget and the supplies, purchased services, and other expenses budget.

FICA. Federal Insurance Contributions Act, commonly known as Social Security.

Fiscal period. Twelve-month period that may or may not coincide with the calendar year. Many organizations use a natural business year, which ends at a time of low business activity. Others may use a year dictated by a closely related governmental unit.

Fixed (forecast) budget. Type of budget, like the appropriation budget, that contains estimates for a single level of activity. Deviations from planned expenditures do not require the same formal actions as the appropriation budget, thus making this type of budget more flexible.

Flexible budget. Budget that takes into account the fact that certain costs vary with the level of activity and other costs remain fixed over a relevant range of activity. Flexible budgets anticipate the possibility of change and show planned revenues and expenses at various levels of activity.

Full-time equivalent. Equivalent of one employee working full-time, that is, 2,080 hours per year. For example, two employees working half-time are one full-time equivalent.

Functional reporting. Reporting of financial information according to type of activity, such as nursing, housekeeping, and dietary. One advantage of this type of reporting is that service costs among hospitals can be compared.

Hill–Burton Act. Hospital Survey and Construction Act of 1949 (Public Law 79-725, Section 60 I et seq.), which allocates federal funds to each state for construction of new beds and for modernization according to a formula based on population and per capita income.

Job control system. Document that lists every approved job position, whether filled or vacant, within each cost center (department). Each position in the document is supported by a detailed job description. The document is used for controlling personnel costs. It is also called a position control system.

Lapsing schedules. Depreciation schedules that show all fixed assets currently in use and their year of acquisition, the costs of the assets, their projected useful lives, the method of depreciation, the rate of depreciation, accumulated depreciation, and the net value of the assets.

Malpractice insurance. *See* **Professional liability insurance.**

Medicaid. State-administered program for providing medical care to the indigent. Federal legislation provides for grants to states to share the financing of the program. Medicaid legislation is officially entitled Grants to States for Medical Assistance

Programs as established by Title XIX of the Social Security Amendments of 1965 (Public Law 89-97) as amended by Public Law 93-233.

Medicare. Federal health insurance program for the aged (over 65) and disabled as established by Title XVIII of the Social Security Amendments of 1965 (Public Law 89-97, which was approved and signed into law July 30, 1965). It also covers dialysis patients suffering from renal failure.

Net income. Amount of net revenue minus operating expenses and nonoperating income and expenses for a given period. Net income is presented as the bottom line of the income statement. Net income provides the necessary funds for working capital, capital, and, for investor-owned institutions, the dividend payments to their shareholders.

Not-for-profit. Term that refers to the tax exemption of certain types of organizations. Those entities are organized under a provision of the federal tax regulations and, in return for meeting a number of specific requirements, do not have to pay tax on net income. The term is often misunderstood and incorrectly thought to refer to an organization that does not require a net income or profit.

Operating budget. Overall plan that identifies the expected resources and expenditures of an entity for a given future period, usually one year. The document defines in monetary terms the policies and plans of the organization and provides a basis for evaluating the financial performance of the plans, controlling costs, and communicating short-range plans and financial requirements within the organization and to the community.

Operating environment. Conditions and circumstances surrounding and affecting the current operations and future development of an organization.

Operating margin. That portion of net income attributable to the excess of operating revenue over operating expenses. The operating margin includes revenue from the coffee shop, cafeteria, gift shop, and medical record reprints. It does not include such items as the gain or loss on the sale of capital assets.

Outpatient. Ambulatory patient who visits the hospital for services but is not admitted to the hospital.

Patient day. Common statistical measurement of hospital activity. A patient day represents one patient in the hospital overnight when the official census is taken.

Patient-day statistics. Data used for making reasonable predictions of overall future demands for service. The daily census report, which reflects the information by nursing unit, is the source of historical patient-day data. For analysis, patient day may be classified by accommodation, payer responsibility, or type of service.

Payer. Person or organization that pays the hospital for services rendered to patients. This can be the patient, an individual guarantor, and/or third parties such as Medicare, Medicaid, Blue Cross, or commercial insurance plans.

Personnel budget. Portion of the expense budget that includes all expenses related to personnel, such as salaries and wages, fringe benefits, premium pay, vacation relief, holiday relief, on-call pay, and shift differentials.

Pooled investments. Assets of two or more accounts or funds consolidated for advantageous investment purposes.

Price master. Schedule that contains the hospital's laboratory and test codes (service codes), the official price relating to that specific service, appropriate account and cost center for each code, description of each code, and technical and professional proportion of the charges.

Professional liability. Obligation of provider to pay for damages resulting from the provider's acts of omission in treating patients. Such financial liability can be covered by professional liability insurance (also called malpractice insurance).

Professional liability insurance. Insurance, also called malpractice insurance, covering the costs of defending suits instituted against the professional and/or any damages assessed by the court. There are two types of professional liability insurance: occurrence policies, in which the insurer is liable for all cases that result from an action that occurred during the policy year, and claims-made policies, in which the insurer is only liable for claims asserted during the policy year regardless of the year in which the action on which the claim is based occurred.

Rate review or rate setting. Process of having an outside party review and approve the hospital budget and the related prices prior to implementation. Rate review is established by legislation or regulations in some states or by contract with certain payers. The process affects the hospital's budget timetable and often its procedures for documentation.

Regulators. Federal, state, and local agencies that attempt to effectively control elements of the hospital industry and audit operations through regulatory legislation. Hospital regulation concerns such issues as capital acquisition, limits on expenditures, access to medical care, and environmental and energy issues.

Relative value units. Indexing technique for relating work effort to output. As a measure of output, relative value units are particularly helpful in determining work load, measuring productivity, or calculating procedure costs in service areas such as the laboratory or the radiology department.

Responsibility accounting. Accounting system that accumulates and communicates revenue, expenses, and statistical data on the basis of established organizational units responsible for producing the revenue and incurring the expenses.

Return-on-equity rates. Net income divided by invested equity. The return-on-equity rates define the amount of net income earned per dollar of equity investment.

Revenue budget. Document that identifies each of the different types of revenue to be earned, according to the period in which it will be earned.

Social Security Act. *See* **FICA.**

Specific-purpose funds. Funds restricted by the donor or by contractual agreement, such as a grant for a specific purpose or project. Board-designated funds do not constitute specific-purpose funds.

Statistical budget. Nonmonetary statistical data relating to the volume and scope of activity in the hospital. Statistical data are essential to both the planning and control stages of budgeting. Examples of data in the statistical budget are number of admissions, patient days of service, percentage of occupancy, and average length of stay.

Step-down distribution. One type of cost-finding technique that involves a series of distributions of the costs of non–revenue-producing departments. When this technique is used, the department that provides services to the greatest number of other departments is closed out first and allocated. The others are closed and allocated in order on the basis of service to other departments.

Strategic plan. Document that identifies the overall direction in which the institution will be moving, that is, where the institution should be many years hence, and its priorities.

Support departments. Departments, also known as general departments, that do not directly generate revenue from patients and are therefore referred to as non–revenue-producing departments.

Tax-exempt institution. *See* **Not-for-profit.**

Third-party payers. Entities such as Medicare, Medicaid, Blue Cross, and commercial insurance companies that contract with individual hospitals and patients to pay for the care of covered patients.

Time studies. Industrial engineering technique used in determining relative value units.

Trend analysis. Management tool that compares a hospital's performance over a given period.

Uniform reporting. Standardized format for reporting financial data. It should not be confused with uniform accounting, which goes beyond the report format and attempts to dictate how each transaction should be recorded. The concept of uniform reporting is becoming popular because it is considered essential for comparing financial statements and ratios within an industry.

Unrestricted funds. Funds that have not been restricted by donor or by contractual arrangements.

Variance analysis. The process of analyzing and evaluating differences between actual and budgeted performance.

Working capital. Hospital's investment in current assets, such as cash, short-term securities, accounts receivable, and inventories. Net working capital is defined as current assets minus current liabilities.

Zero-based budget. Budgeting method by which the hospital manager must annually reevaluate all activities to decide whether they should be eliminated or funded. Appropriate funding levels are then determined by priorities and ranking established by top management according to the overall availability of funds.

Index

Accountability, 1–2
Accounting costs, 8
Admissions, 68; estimates of, 87–89
American Hospital Association, *Chart of Accounts for Hospitals*, 112–13, 122
Ancillary department statistics, 93
Appropriation budgets, 31
Association dues, 126

Balance sheet, 151–52; and change in financial position, 78, 154; sources of figures in, 152–53
Basic responsibility reporting, 35–37
Bed complement statistic, 86–87
Biweekly payroll reports, 160, 161
Blue Cross plans, contracting under, 53–54; payment policies of, 129–30
Budget, 3, 15; definition of, 3; format and guidelines for, 67; linking of, to long-term goals, 17; methods of reviewing, 4; operating expense in, 72; period of, 23–24, 63; preliminary revenue in, 71; tentative, 73–74. *See also* Budget process; Capital budget; Cash budget; Operating budget; Projected financial statements
Budget calendar, 64
Budget committee, 61–62, 73; approval of operating budget by, 75
Budget director, 85
Budgeted costs, 8
Budget package, as communication tool, 3–4
Budget period, 63
Budget process, 61–62; budget committee approval in, 75; budget format and guidelines in, 67; budget period for, 23–24, 63; cash availability and, 74; changes in, 1; department activity level in, 70; description of current operations and environment in, 63; detailed personnel budget in, 71–72; determination of desired net income in, 74; final approval of, 75; and long-range planning, 67; and new and upgraded position requests and proposed position eliminations, 72–73; and operating expense budget, 72; and organizational structure, 63; policies, goals, and objectives in, 62; and preliminary revenue budget, 71; and preparations for budgeting, 62; and program addition, modification, or elimination, 73, 75; and rate increases, 75; and reporting system, 63–64; role of management in, 61; role of medical staff management in, 61; and scale and merit salary increases, 74; and staffing levels, 70–71; and tentative budget, 73; and volume forecasts for emergency department visits, 69–70; and volume forecasts for patient days, 67–69; work sheet package used in, 64–67. *See also* Planning, budgeting, and managing process

Cafeteria revenue, 107, 131
Capital, sources of, 141
Capital budget, 3, 27, 141–43; and capital expenditure requests, 143–48; role of strategic planning in, 141
Capital expenditure requests, 143–48
Capital projects, funding for, 143